MCQs IN PAEDIATRICS

MCQs in Paediatrics

J. M. Gupta, MD, FRCPE, FRACP, D.Ch
Associate Professor of Paediatrics
University of New South Wales, Australia

and

J. Beveridge, FRACP
Emiritus Professor of Paediatrics
University of New South Wales, Australia

With a Foreword by

Hans Henning Bode, MD, FRACP
Head, School of Paediatrics, University of New South Wales,
Clinical Director, Prince of Wales Children's Hospital, Australia

CHAPMAN & HALL MEDICAL
London · Glasgow · New York · Tokyo · Melbourne · Madras

Published by Chapman & Hall, 2-6 Boundary Row, London SE1 8HN

Chapman & Hall, 2-6 Boundary Row, London SE1 8HN, UK

Blackie Academic & Professional, Wester Cleddens Road, Bishopbriggs, Glasgow G64 2NZ, UK

Chapman & Hall GmbH, Pappelallee 3, 69469 Weinheim, Germany

Chapman & Hall USA, One Penn Plaza, 41st Floor, New York, NY10119, USA

Chapman & Hall Japan, ITP - Japan, Kyowa Building, 3F, 2-2-1 Hirakawacho, Chiyoda-ku, Tokyo 102, Japan

Chapman & Hall Australia, Thomas Nelson Australia, 102 Dodds Street, South Melbourne, Victoria 3205, Australia

Chapman & Hall India, R. Seshadri, 32 Second Main Road, CIT East, Madras 600 035, India

First edition 1993
Reprinted 1993, 1994, 1995

© 1993 J.M. Gupta and J. Beveridge

Typeset in Great Britain by Acorn Bookwork, Salisbury, Wiltshire
Printed in Great Britain by Page Bros (Norwich) Ltd

ISBN 0 412 48310 6

A Catalogue record for this book is available from the British Library

Library of Congress Cataloging-in-Publication Data available

∞ Printed on acid-free paper, manufactured in accordance with ANSI/NISO Z39.48-1992 and ANSI/NISO Z39.48-1984 (Permanence of Paper)

Contents

Preface

Multiple choice question examinations have become the accepted norm for assessment of undergraduate and postgraduate students because they are considered to test a wide range of topics, easier to mark and provide objectivity. The marks awarded do not depend on the whims, moods and fancies of the examiners. Computer analysis of the results allows rapid processing of large numbers of candidates and produces results within a short time of the collection of papers. The statistical analysis of the performance of the paper as a whole as well as the performance of good students compared to those of poor students allows planning of further strategies in teaching. However, the setting of these questions requires a considerable amount of work prior to the examination in order to avoid ambiguity and personal bias of the examiners.

At the University of New South Wales, the School of Paediatrics has used multiple choice questions for more than 15 years. The questions were supplied by the staff of the School and the Prince of Wales Children's Hospital. The questions were scrutinized by an examination committee and their suitability was tested by computer analysis of the results. Over this period we have accumulated more than 1000 questions. The questions in this book were selected from this bank of questions. More questions were added in subject areas which were felt to be deficient.

The critiques were written with the aim of stimulating the student to think rather than simply recall information. Additional information is provided which facilitates further learning and problem-solving abilities.

It would be obvious that this book would have been impossible to produce without the tremendous amount of work put in by our colleagues at the School of Paediatrics, University of New South Wales and Prince of Wales Children's Hospital to whom we are extremely grateful. Unfortunately space does not permit us to thank them individually. We would also like to acknowledge the help of our secretaries, Lillan Holgate and Liz Noakes, for preparing the manu-script and Professor H.H. Bode for writing the foreword.

J.M. GUPTA
J. BEVERIDGE

Foreword

During the past 40 years paediatrics as a specialty in medicine has made enormous advances and expanded into subspecialties representing almost all aspects of medicine. A vast body of new knowledge has been accumulated and many new avenues have been opened for research and clinical application. The revolutionary advances in basic science during the past four decades, especially those in molecular biology, physics and immunology have led to the development of diagnostic and therapeutic tools which were beyond the imagination of even the most optimistic and farsighted clinician four decades ago. No longer can we expect students to digest the enormous wealth of knowledge in Paediatrics. Indeed, specialization within the academic faculty has become so detailed as to endanger the training in general paediatrics and the preparation of medical students for internship and general practice.

The authors of this book were keenly aware of this peril. They deserve to be commended for compiling a volume of questions which addresses general paediatric knowledge and clinical skills rather than memory of highly specialized or esoteric facts.

Professor Gupta and Professor Beveridge share a long and distinguished career in paediatric education and have made many innovative contributions to the teaching of child health. John Beveridge achieved prominence in medicine reaching well beyond Australia. He was the first paediatrician appointed to the Board of Censors of the Royal Australasian College of Physicians and served with such distinction that his colleagues entrusted him with the establishment of a separate paediatric training programme recognizing the similarities to adult medicine as well as the significant differences. As the Foundation Professor of Paediatrics at the University of New South Wales and Clinical Director of the Prince of Wales Children's Hospital he established a very successful training programme for students and paediatric house staff. Much of the support for these programmes was provided by Professor Jagdish Gupta who joined the School of Paediatrics at the University of New

South Wales after accumulating extensive teaching and research experience abroad. Together they also initiated special Diploma and Masters programmes in the School of Paediatrics. These programmes are still unique in Australia and have achieved very prestigious status.

The text of this book is divided into fifteen chapters representing the various developmental aspects and subspecialties of paediatrics. Questions are listed in groups of five, the answers are conveniently provided on the reverse side of the page. It is highly commendable that comments on each question are provided, rather than indications only for the correct answers. The questions have been carefully selected and worded, then subjected to rigorous critical reviews by the various faculties, resulting in a useful gauge that discriminates between students of greater and lesser knowledge.

This book provides a very valuable aid to the evaluation of students and of teaching programmes. The questions should not and are not intended to be used as the sole method of student evaluation. However, in conjunction with carefully designed clinical examination these questions have been judged to be valuable and to provide a fair assessment of competence by the teaching faculty as well as by the student bodies to whom they were presented.

Hans Henning Bode

1 Growth and development

1.1. Compared to the body proportions of a 5-year-old child, the newborn infant has

A   a larger head.
B   a larger liver.
C   shorter extremities.
D   a larger mandible.
E   smaller tonsils.

1.2. When compared with the body proportions of an adult, an infant has

A   a larger head.
B   longer legs.
C   a longer trunk.
D   an increased upper segment to lower segment body ratio.
E   a larger arm span.

1.3. In regard to growth during gestation

A   babies born at 38 weeks' gestation weigh more at birth on average, than those born after 40 weeks' gestation.
B   size at birth correlates better with maternal stature than paternal stature.
C   hormonal influences on growth are independent of fetal sex.
D   the peak increase in fetal weight occurs during the third trimester.
E   twins achieve their maximum weight velocity by 32 weeks' gestation.

1.4. Which of the following statements is/are correct?

A   Babies are able to respond to sounds in utero.
B   Full-term babies are unable to follow a large object at birth with their eyes.
C   A 6-week-old infant would be able to follow a large object through an arc of 135°.
D   Growth velocity of head decreases with age.
E   A 12-month-old infant who keeps falling when starting to walk is likely to have cerebral palsy.

1.1. A B C E
Compared to the body proportions of a 5-year-old child, the newborn infant has a larger head, larger liver and short extremities. The mandible has the same proportions though it is smaller compared to a pubescent child. Lymphoid tissue (including tonsils) grows from birth to puberty and then involutes.

1.2. A C D
Compared to an adult, an infant has a larger head, shorter limbs and a longer trunk. As a result it has an increased upper segment to lower segment body ratio and a smaller arm span.

1.3. A B C D E
After the age of 40 weeks' gestation, the placenta develops infarcts and is unable to maintain adequate nutrition of the infant. Epidemiological studies have shown that size at birth correlates better with maternal than paternal stature. There is very little production of testosterone in fetal life and therefore it has no effect on fetal growth. During the last trimester of pregnancy the fetus gains in weight because of deposition of fat. It has been shown that weight velocity decreases after the 'litter' has achieved a certain weight which is at 32 weeks' gestation for twins.

1.4. A C D
Babies respond to sound in utero as demonstrated by changes in heart rate. At birth full-term babies will follow a human face or a large red ball with their eyes. A 6-week-old infant will follow a large object through an arc of 180°. Head growth is maximum in the first year of life and decreases progressively thereafter. Infants tend to keep falling when learning to walk.

1.5. Compared with older children, full-term infants at 1 month have
A a higher risk of gram-negative infections.
B a smaller risk of iron deficiency anaemia.
C higher fluid requirements per kilogram of body weight.
D a smaller surface area per kilogram of body weight.
E a larger head size compared to body length.

1.6. A 4-week-old infant
A usually has a social smile.
B is able to lift head momentarily in prone position.
C needs 20 hours of sleep.
D has a Moro reflex.
E can hold a rattle.

1.7. A normal 4-week-old infant
A is in danger of suffocation if nursed prone.
B will follow a small light through an arc of 180°.
C will regard the human face.
D can distinguish his mother from other people.
E will follow a large object to the midline.

1.8. A 6-week-old infant
A will roll over.
B puts out his arms to be picked up.
C is able to turn his head towards a loud noise.
D will regard the human face.
E holds his head up momentarily in the prone position.

1.5.   A B C E

Compared with older children, infants at 1 month have higher risk of gram-negative infections because they do not have any maternal or acquired immunity against these organisms, are at no risk of iron deficiency anaemia (unless there has been bleeding) because of iron stores derived from the mother, need higher fluid requirements per kg of body weight because of higher metabolic rate. Their surface area per kg of their body weight is higher and their head is larger compared to their body length.

1.6.   B D

Infants do not usually smile till the age of 6 weeks and do not have any set pattern of sleep. At 4 weeks they are able to lift their head momentarily in the prone position and have a complete Moro reflex. They are unable to hold a rattle because of the presence of the grasp reflex.

1.7.   C E

In the prone position a 4-week-old infant is at no risk of suffocation as it will be able to lift its head and turn to the side. Though such an infant will follow a large object through an arc of 180°, it will not be able to do so with a small light. The infant is attracted by the human face (this may be a diagram on a cardboard) but does not distinguish between different people.

1.8.   D E

A 6-week-old infant will follow a human face through an arc of 180° but not a small light, will not put out his arms to be picked up till the age of 5 months and is unable to turn his head towards a loud noise though he may show evidence of hearing. In the prone position the infant can hold his head up momentarily.

1.9. By the age of 4 months most infants
A   can roll over.
B   have conjugate eye movements.
C   reach out and grab objects.
D   sit with support.
E   have two incisor teeth.

1.10. Which of the following developmental attainments is/are appropriate for a full-term infant at the age of 6 months?
A   Sits but needs to be propped.
B   Reaches with a strong hand preference.
C   Fixes but does not follow a moving face.
D   When placed prone on a table lifts his head and supports the upper trunk on extended arms.
E   Has a brisk, symmetrical Moro response.

1.11. In which of the following conditions are infantile body proportions seen in a 5-year-old child?
A   Malnutrition.
B   Osteogenesis imperfecta.
C   Untreated congenital hypothyroidism.
D   Achondroplasia.
E   Down's syndrome.

1.12. A 30-week (7-month)-old infant would be expected to
A   transfer an object from one hand to the other.
B   be toilet trained.
C   clap hands in imitation.
D   be distressed by the approach of strangers.
E   be able to sit up.

1.9. A B C

By the age of 4 months most infants can roll over, have conjugate eye movements and can reach out and grab small objects. They do not sit with support till the age of 5 months and do not have incisor teeth till the age of 5–7 months.

1.10. A D

A normal full-term 6-month-old infant is able to sit with support and lift his head and support the upper trunk on extended arms. He shows no hand preference. The Moro reflex disappears by the age of 5 months. By the age of 6 weeks most children will be able to fix and follow a moving face.

1.11. B C D

In achondroplasia and congenital hypothyroidism there is abnormality of the epiphyseal centres which results in diminution of linear growth of long bones. As a result the infantile body proportions (crown pubis/crown heel: 1.7/1) are maintained. In malnutrition there is delay in growth of ossification centres but there is no disturbance of epiphyseal growth. In Down's syndrome the body proportions are normal. In osteogenesis imperfecta there may be shortening of limbs because of fractures.

1.12. A E

A 7-month-old infant is able to transfer an object from one hand to the other and is able to sit up. Toilet training is variable but is seldom below the age of 2 years. Infants clap hands at the age of 8–9 months and are not distressed by the approach of strangers till the age of 7–8 months.

1.13. Which of the following skills would be expected of a 7-month-old infant but not of a 5-month-old infant?

A   Crawls.
B   Smiles socially.
C   Controls his bowel and bladder.
D   Sits unsupported.
E   Raises his head while prone.

1.14. An 8-month-old infant

A   has thumb–finger grasp.
B   bounces actively when held up.
C   is able to control his bowel and bladder.
D   sits unsupported.
E   uses 'Mama' and/or 'Dada' meaningfully.

1.15. Inability to do which of the following would be of concern in a baby of 9 months?

A   Sit unaided.
B   Use words with meaning.
C   Use pincer grip.
D   Put food in the mouth.
E   Change objects from one hand to the other.

1.16. Which of the following developmental attainments is/are appropriate for a child of 10 months?

A   Has good finger–thumb apposition with the left hand but uses a mild palmar grasp on the right.
B   Crawls symmetrically by dragging his extended legs behind, using his forearms.
C   Has a symmetrical forward parachute reaction.
D   Responds to noise but cannot localize the source.
E   Is mobile by shuffling along on his bottom in a sitting position.

1.13. D
Both 5- and 7-month-old infants will smile and raise their head while prone, will not crawl or be able to control their bowel and bladder. The 7-month-old would be able to sit unsupportedly whereas the 5-month-old will not.

1.14. B D
Thumb–finger grasp and control of bowel and bladder would not occur in an 8-month-old infant. He bounces when held up and babbles but does not use words meaningfully.

1.15. A D E
More than 90% of children at the age of 9 months will be able to sit up unaided, put food in their mouth and transfer objects from one hand to the other. Pincer grip and words of meaning do not develop till the age of 10 months in most infants.

1.16. C E
A 10-month-old infant should have good finger–thumb apposition on both hands, crawl without dragging his legs, has a symmetrical parachute reaction, is able to localize sounds and can move around by crawling.

1.17. A 10-month-old infant differs from a 3-month-old infant in his ability to

A   sit unsupported.
B   use pincer grip to pick up a raisin.
C   control his bowel and bladder.
D   crawl.
E   raise his head while prone.

1.18. Which of the following is/are likely in a 10-month-old child who plays with his urine or stool?

A   Retarded.
B   Emotionally disturbed.
C   Autistic.
D   Normal.
E   Spoilt.

1.19. Which of the following is/are true?

A   A 4-month-old infant is unlikely to produce vocal sounds other than crying.
B   An 8-month-old infant can hold his head steady in the sitting position.
C   A 6-month-old infant can be toilet-trained.
D   It is normal for a 9-month-old child to have no aversion to play in his urine or stool.
E   A 1-year-old child would be expected to give up a toy on request.

1.20. A 1-year-old child would be expected to

A   uncover an object (which was covered before the infant could grasp it).
B   grasp a raisin.
C   play simple ball game.
D   feed himself a biscuit.
E   put three words together.

1.17. A B D
Both 10- and 3-month-old infants are unable to control their bowel and bladder and are able to raise their head while prone. A 10-month-old infant is able to sit unsupported, use a pincer grip and crawl in contrast to a 3-month-old infant.

1.18. D
It is normal for 10-month-old children to play with their urine or stool.

1.19. B D E
A 4-month-old infant would babble. Infants are able to hold their heads steady in the sitting position by the age of 3–4 months. Toilet training (as distinct from anticipation or 'reflex' training) cannot be achieved till the infant is able to voluntarily contract the anal sphincter and verbalize his needs. At the age of 8 months children have not developed the ability to distinguish between being clean and dirty. Children achieve the ability to give up a toy on request by the age of 8–9 months.

1.20. A B C D
At 15 months a child can make a tower of two cubes and at 2 years a tower of four to six cubes. At 9–10 months, infants can grasp a raisin, feed a biscuit and uncover an object covered in their presence. They can play simple ball games by the age of 1 year. They are usually unable to put three words together till the age of 2 years.

1.21. Ninety percent of children at 1 year would

A   build a tower of three cubes.
B   have a well developed pincer grip.
C   give up a toy on request.
D   walk without support.
E   show stranger anxiety.

1.22. Which of the following behaviours are observed in a child at 12 months but not at 8 months of age?

A   Stands alone well.
B   Makes postural adjustments to dressing.
C   Walks up steps.
D   Finger–thumb grasp.
E   Combines two words.

1.23. An infant aged 16 months was referred for assessment of suspected mental retardation. Which of the following findings is/are outside the range of normal?

A   He does not scribble spontaneously with pencil on paper.
B   He does not walk alone.
C   'Ma' and 'Dada' are the only words which are clearly recognizable.
D   He is unable to build a tower of four cubes.
E   He is unable to throw an object.

1.24. The majority of children at age 18 months are expected to be able to

A   sit steadily on the floor unaided.
B   say ten words.
C   make a tower of three blocks when shown.
D   find a toy under a cup.
E   chew a biscuit.

11

1.21. B C E
More than 90% of children at 1 year would have a well-developed pincer grip which is usually present at the age of 10 months, give up a toy on request and show stranger anxiety (usually present at 7–8 months). Most infants will not be able to build a tower of three cubes till the age of 18 months and walk without support till the age of 15 months.

1.22. A B D
In contrast to children at 8 months, children at 12 months are able to stand alone, make postural adjustments to dressing and have a well-developed pincer grip. They are unable to walk up steps or combine two words.

1.23. E
Children do not scribble till the age of 2 years. Not all children would walk alone by the age of 16 months. Many children at 16 months have a lot of jargon but may only have a few recognizable words. A child of 16 months is not expected to make a tower of more than three cubes but is able to throw an object.

1.24. A B C D E
At the age of 18 months the majority of children have a vocabulary of 10 words and make a tower of 3 blocks. They can sit up alone without support and chew a biscuit by the age of 9–10 months. They can find a toy under a cup at the age of 10 months.

1.25. Inability to do which of the following in a 20-month child is a cause for concern?

A   Speak in clear two to three word phrases.
B   Walk unaided.
C   Kick a ball.
D   Build a tower of eight blocks.
E   Cooperate with dressing.

1.26. A 2-year-old child should be able to

A   name three colours correctly.
B   use plurals.
C   build a tower of five blocks.
D   kick a ball on request.
E   hop on one foot.

1.27. By 2 years of age most children

A   are talking in three word sentences.
B   are able to use a knife and fork.
C   know their surname.
D   can hop and skip.
E   can copy on paper squares and crosses.

1.28. Most developmentally normal infants of 2 years

A   are able to kick a ball without falling.
B   can name three colours.
C   can ride a tricycle.
D   can build a tower of six blocks.
E   can use the past tense in speech.

1.25. B E

More than 90% of children at the age of 20 months will be able to walk unaided and cooperate with dressing. Ability to put eight blocks together is not achieved till the age of 30 months and the ability to put three words together is achieved at the age of 36 months.

1.26. C D

Children can name three to four colours correctly at the age of 5 years, use plurals at the age of 3 years and hop at the age of 4 years. They can build a tower of four to six blocks and kick a ball on request at the age of 2 years.

1.27. A

By the age of 2 years most children are able to put a subject, verb and object together, use a spoon (not knife and fork), know their first name but not surname. Children cannot hop and skip till the age of 4 years.

1.28. A D

Children at 2 years can kick a ball without falling and build a tower of six blocks. They can name three colours by the age of 5 years and ride a tricycle at 3 years. They can use the past tense in speech at the age of 30–36 months.

1.29. Which of the following statements is/are true?
A Most infants can chew at 3 months.
B The normal respiratory rate of a 1-year-old child is between 20 and 30/ min.
C A 2-year-old child is 'self centred'.
D The average blood pressure of a 3-year-old child is 120/80.
E A 5-year-old child is able to copy a circle.

1.30. Which of the following conditions is/are within the normal range of development at 4 years of age?
A Faecal soiling.
B Day wetting.
C Thumb sucking.
D Occasional masturbation.
E Night wetting.

1.31. A 5-year-old child should be able to
A draw a man (with body, head, etc.).
B identify four colours.
C copy a circle.
D count from 100 backwards.
E skip with alternate feet.

1.32. The majority of 6-year-old children would be expected to be able to
A hop on one foot.
B draw a recognizable picture of a man and include the head.
C define justice and honesty.
D identify his right and left arms.
E tie his shoelaces.

15

1.29. B C E

Infants are unable to carry the food to the back of the mouth with the tongue before the age of 4 months. At birth the normal respiratory rate is 40–60 per minute and it drops gradually till it is 20–30 per minute at the age of 1 year. By the age of 18 months the respiratory rate is between 15 and 25 per minute. Children at 2 years do not 'share' their possessions and tend to play in 'parallel' rather than participate in games. At birth the infant's blood pressure is 80/50 and it progressively increases throughout life. Adult values (120/80) are not reached till the age of 16 years. Most children are able to copy a circle by the age of 5 years.

1.30. C D E

Thumb sucking, occasional masturbation and teeth grinding are normal for a child of 4 years. Most children are dry by day and do not have faecal soiling by this age.

1.31. A B C E

A 5-year-old child will be able to draw a man (with body, head and four or five parts), identify four colours, copy a circle and skip. He will be able to count up to ten.

1.32. A B D E

Children can hop on one foot at the age of 5 years, draw a recognizable picture of a man with two to four parts other than the head at the age of 4 years, identify right and left arms and tie their shoelaces at the age of 6 years. They do not conceptualize abstract terms like justice and honesty till the age of 8–10 years.

1.33. Which of the following statement(s) is/are true?

A An adolescent goitre is usually associated with hyperthyroidism.
B The early development of breast tissue in pubescent females is often unilateral.
C In girls the adolescent growth spurt follows the menarche by approximately 1 year.
D There has been a decrease in the age of menarche over the past century.
E The first sign of pubertal development in boys is growth of facial hair.

1.34. Which of the following problems are more likely to be found in adolescents compared to children under 12 years old?

A Recurrent abdominal pain.
B Crohn's disease.
C Intussusception.
D Conduct disorder.
E Acne.

1.35. Which of the following statements about puberty is/are correct?

A The peak height velocity usually occurs following the onset of menstruation in girls.
B There is an increase in androgen secretion at puberty in girls.
C The pituitary hormone which stimulates hormonal activity by the gonads is the same in both sexes.
D The average peak height velocity occurs at an earlier age in girls than in boys.
E The average peak height velocity is less in girls than in boys.

1.36. Which of the following statements is/are true of sexual development at puberty?

A Sexual maturation is more closely correlated with bone maturation than with chronological age.
B Girls mature earlier than boys.
C Testicular enlargement is the first sign of puberty in boys.
D Breast hypertrophy is rare (less than 10%) in boys at puberty.
E During the first year following menarche, the menstrual periods of most girls are anovulatory.

1.33. B D
Breast development is usually asymmetrical and may cause anxiety to pre-pubescent girls. The adolescent growth spurt occurs prior to menarche. The decrease in the age of menarche is thought to be due to better nutrition. The first sign of pubertal development in boys is the increase in size of the testes.

1.34. B D E
Recurrent abdominal pains are more likely to occur in children below the age of 12. Intussusception most commonly occurs in infants aged 6–9 months. Crohn's disease, conduct disorder and acne are more likely to be found in adolescents than in children under 12 years old.

1.35. B C D E
The peak height velocity in girls is at the onset of puberty which is well before the onset of menstruation. In girls as well as in boys increased androgen secretion by the adrenal gland is responsible for the development of pubic and axillary hair. The follicle-stimulating hormone (FSH) stimulates the production of testosterone and oestrogen. The peak height velocity in girls is at 12–14 years as compared to 12.5–15 years in boys. However, the average peak height velocity is less in girls than in boys because of the earlier onset of their growth spurt.

1.36. A B C E
Bone and sexual maturation are both under the control of androgens and may not have any correlation to chronological age. On the average girls mature one to two years earlier than boys. Testicular enlargement is the first sign of puberty in boys. Breast hypertrophy is common in boys. At puberty following menarche menstrual periods are anovulatory in the first year in most girls.

1.37. Which of the following has/have an increased incidence in adolescence?
A   Thyrotoxicosis.
B   Acne vulgaris.
C   Peptic ulceration.
D   Anorexia nervosa.
E   Scoliosis.

1.38. A head circumference measurement falling on the 10th percentile for a given age indicates that
A   ten percent of the normal children of the same age would have the same measurement.
B   the patient's head circumference is 10% below the mean value for the age.
C   the patient's head circumference is 10% above the lower limit of the normal range.
D   ten per cent of normal children of the same age would have a greater measurement than the patient in question.
E   ten per cent of normal children of the same age would have the same or lower measurement.

1.39. A 10-month-old male child who at 5 months was on the 50th percentile for height, weight and head circumference is now still on the 50th percentile for height and weight but is above the 97th percentile for head circumference. Which of the following statements is/are true?
A   It is not of concern if either parent's head circumference is on or above the 97th percentile.
B   The parents can be reassured as the head circumference is within normal range.
C   He ought to be reviewed in 6 months.
D   The head circumference should be measured again and checked.
E   The child should be referred for specialist assessment.

1.40. Which of the following statements is/are true of a child aged 8 months whose length lies on the 10th percentile and whose head circumference lies on the 10th percentile?
A   He is abnormally short and should be investigated.
B   He is likely to be normal.
C   He is suffering from microcephaly.
D   He is at least as long as 10 in every 100 children of his age.
E   He is failing to thrive.

1.37. A B D E
The peak incidence of thyrotoxicosis is in adolescence. At puberty increased levels of androgens result in increase in size and secretions of sebaceous follicles resulting in acne. Anorexia nervosa and scoliosis have their onset in early puberty and have an increased incidence in girls. There is no evidence that incidence of peptic ulceration is increased at puberty.

1.38. E
When quantitative measurements are arranged in order of ascending magnitude, the percentile points refer to values falling on or below that centile.

1.39. D E
Children may have large heads because their parents' head sizes are large. Even though the head circumference is normal for some children, it is abnormal for this child as it has crossed centiles while the weight and height have remained on the same centiles. The head circumference should be measured again to ensure that the measurement is correct. If it is correct, specialist referral is indicated. Frequent review (fortnightly or monthly) is mandatory.

1.40. B D
As this child's head circumference and length fall on the same centiles the child does not require any investigations for 'short stature'. The child's head circumference is normal for his length. The 10th percentile means that 10% of the children have the same length or less than this child. Without knowing the weight of the child it is incorrect to say he is 'failing to thrive'.

1.41. Gynaecomastia in boys is significantly associated with
A   obesity.
B   Klinefelter's syndrome.
C   Noonan's syndrome.
D   cirrhosis of liver.
E   feminizing tumour of adrenals.

1.42. Which of the following statements is/are true of brain growth?
A   There is a period of rapid postnatal growth of the cerebellum during the first year of life.
B   The size of the brain is at 50% of adult size at 5 years of age.
C   There is no growth from increase in cell number after birth.
D   There is little growth from increase in number of neurons after 12 months postnatal age.
E   Cell number and cell connections increase in parallel during growth of the brain.

1.43. Which of the following statements is/are true of skeletal growth?
A   The change from infantile to mature facial proportions is due to the more rapid growth of the upper part of the facial skeleton, compared with the lower part.
B   Elongation of long bones in childhood and adolescence occurs mainly at the primary ossification centres.
C   Relative to ossified bone, the amount of cartilage in bone increases with maturity.
D   High dose androgens accelerate bone maturation (e.g. epiphyseal fusion) more rapidly than linear growth.
E   The lower femoral epiphyses are evident on X-ray before the upper femoral epiphyses.

1.44. Skeletal proportions are normal in
A   pituitary dwarfism.
B   achondroplasia.
C   delayed adolescence.
D   congential hypothyroidism.
E   emotional deprivation.

1.41. B D E

In obesity and Noonan's syndrome there is no gynaecomastia. In Klinefelter's syndrome there is deficiency of androgen and gynaecomastia. Oestrogens are responsible for the causation of gynaecomastia in cirrhosis of the liver (failure of metabolization of oestrogens) and feminizing tumour of adrenals (excessive oestrogen production by the adrenal gland).

1.42. A D

During the first year of life cerebellum grows rapidly. Brain growth is almost adult size by the age of 5 years. The brain of the term infant contains the full adult component of neurons. In the first year increase in size of brain is the result of myelination, elaboration of neuronal processes (both neurons and dendrites) and of increase in glial cells. Subsequently it is mainly due to elaboration of neuronal processes.

1.43. D E

The mandible grows faster than the rest of the face at puberty. Elongation of long bones occurs both at primary and secondary ossification centres. With maturity the cartilage is replaced by ossified bone. Androgens accelerate bone maturation and stimulate osteogenesis which results in epiphyseal fusion and ultimate diminution of linear growth. The lower femoral epiphysis is present at birth whereas the upper femoral epiphysis appears in the first year of life.

1.44. A C E

In achondroplasia and cretinism the limbs grow slowly because of epiphyseal dysplasia. In delayed adolescence growth of long bones continues for a longer period resulting in normal body proportions. In pituitary dwarfism and emotional deprivation there is lack of growth hormone and body proportions remain normal.

1.45. The anterior fontanelle
A   usually closes by 3 months of age.
B   is rarely pulsatile.
C   marks the junction of the sagittal and coronal sutures.
D   may not bulge in the presence of meningitis.
E   is usually smaller than the posterior fontanelle.

1.46. Delayed eruption of teeth can occur in
A   rickets.
B   severe neonatal hyperbilirubinaemia.
C   hypothyroidism.
D   cleidocranial dysostosis.
E   ectodermal dysplasia.

1.47. Which of the following statements concerning teething is/are correct?
A   A 1-year-old infant is likely to have six to eight deciduous teeth.
B   First deciduous tooth to erupt is upper central incisor.
C   There are 20 deciduous teeth.
D   One of the first permanent teeth to erupt is the lower central incisor.
E   Calcificaton of the first permanent molars begins at birth in a full-term
  - infant.

1.48. Retardation of bone age is a recognized feature of
A   obesity.
B   malabsorption.
C   congential adrenal cortical hyperplasia.
D   isolated growth hormone deficiency.
E   psychosocial deprivation.

1.45. C D

The anterior fontanelle usually closes between 9 and 18 months. It is pulsatile and marks the junction of the sagittal and coronal sutures. It is larger than the posterior fontanelle. Though a bulging fontanelle is seen with meningitis, it may not be present in newborn infants and infants with dehydration.

1.46. A C D

Delayed eruption of the teeth occurs in hypothyroidism, rickets and cleido-cranial dysostosis. Severe neonatal hyperbilirubinaemia causes blue to black discoloration of teeth. In ectodermal dysplasia, the teeth are totally or partially absent.

1.47. A C D E

There is great variability in dental eruption. By the age of 1 year most children will have six to eight teeth. Usually the first tooth to erupt is the lower central incisor. There are 20 deciduous teeth. The first permanent tooth to erupt is the first molar or lower central incisor which occurs at 6–7 years of age. Calcification of first permanent molar begins at birth in a term infant.

1.48. B D E

Bone age is retarded in malabsorption, growth hormone deficiency and psychosocial deprivation. It is accelerated in obesity and in congenital adrenal cortical hyperplasia. In the latter it is due to increased androgen production.

1.49. During growth and development

A thyroid hormone plays an essential part in the maturation of tissues.
B 'bone age' correlates more closely with 'height age' than with 'weight age'.
C the testes are usually in the scrotum by the end of the fourth month of fetal life.
D the earliest sign of puberty in a boy is enlargement of the testes.
E menarche occurs with onset of breast development at puberty.

1.50. Compared with girls, boys

A have a higher infant mortality.
B exhibit the adolescent growth spurt earlier.
C are more likely to have microspherocytosis.
D are more likely to be accidentally drowned.
E pass their milestones of infant development earlier.

1.51. Development of speech in an infant can be delayed by

A late eruption of teeth.
B tongue tie.
C emotional deprivation.
D enlarged adenoids.
E deafness.

1.52. Which of the following statements is/are correct?

A Isolated delay in speech development is an indication to test hearing.
B Presence of babbling does not exclude deafness.
C Tongue tie is a common cause of delayed speech.
D Girls tend to speak at an earlier age than boys.
E Delay in speech development is often familial.

1.49. A B D

Thyroid hormone plays an important part in maturation of tissues in periods of rapid growth. Bone age correlates more closely with height age than with weight age. The testes are in the scrotum by 32–34 weeks' gestation. The earliest sign of puberty in a boy is enlargement of the testes. The onset of menarche occurs much later than breast development at puberty.

1.50. A D

Compared with girls, boys have a higher mortality at all ages. They exhibit the adolescent growth spurt later and are more likely to be accidentally drowned. The inheritance of microspherocytosis is autosomal dominant and there is no difference in incidence between the two sexes. The infant developmental milestones are similar in both sexes.

1.51. C E

Late speech can result from emotional deprivation and deafness. It has no relationship to late eruption of teeth or tongue tie. Enlarged adenoids might distort speech and nasal intonation.

1.52. A B D E

Isolated delay in speech development may be due to loss of hearing. Babbling occurs irrespective of hearing but does not progress to recognizable speech in deaf children. Tongue tie does not cause delayed speech though it may cause indistinct speech. Girls tend to speak at an earlier age than boys. Delay in speech development is often familial.

1.53. A congenitally deaf but intelligent child of 4 years would show which of the following?
A   If he can speak his voice will have metallic and monotonous quality.
B   Communication by gesture.
C   Purposeless play.
D   Frustration tantrums.
E   Clumsiness and incoordination.

1.54. Delay in language development is common in
A   autism.
B   deafness.
C   elective mutism.
D   twins.
E   gross emotional deprivation.

1.55. In normal language development
A   babbling ceases at 6–9 months.
B   vocabulary at 2 years usually comprises about 25–30 words.
C   construction of short sentences is achieved by one year.
D   pronouns are used from 18 months.
E   construction of complex sentences is achieved by 4 years.

1.56. If a 3-year-old male child is not speaking clearly nor making sentences
A   he should have his hearing tested.
B   his speech function could be within normal limits.
C   the child has a 90% chance of being mentally retarded.
D   he should not attend a day-care centre until his speech is improved.
E   the amount of stimulation to speak should be assessed.

1.53. A B D
A congenitally deaf but intelligent child of 4 years would not have purposeless play or show clumsiness and incoordination. If he speaks at all he would have a monotonous voice. He communicates by gesture and is frustrated because of his inability to communicate.

1.54. A B D E
Delay in language development is a feature of autism and gross emotional deprivation. Deafness results in delay in language development because of inability to hear. Twins tend to speak later than singletons because they can communicate with each other and have no need to speak. In elective mutism language development is not delayed.

1.55. B E
Babbling persists till the age of 12 months or later. By the age of 18 months the child has a vocabulary of 50 words. Construction of short sentences (subject, verb, object) is not achieved till the age of 2 years. Children begin to refer to self with the pronoun 'I' or 'me' by the age of 15 months. By 4 years, children are able to construct complex sentences, e.g. relative clauses.

1.56. A B E
Hearing loss is a common cause for unclear speech as the child does not hear the words correctly. Children who have things done for them or can have their needs met by pointing to things, generally do not speak in sentences. Such children benefit by attending a day-care centre as a result of stimulation. Delay in speech may be the presenting symptom of mental retardation; however, many 3-year-old normal children will not have clear speech.

2 Nutrition

2.1. Breast milk production is likely to be increased by
A   extra water in the mother's diet.
B   a strongly sucking infant.
C   extra milk in the mother's diet.
D   administration of stilboestrol.
E   maximal emptying of the breasts.

2.2. Human colostrum compared to mature human milk
A   has higher fat content.
B   has fewer cellular elements.
C   is richer in secretory IgA.
D   contains more protein.
E   has lower water content (%).

2.3. In comparison to human milk, pasteurized cow's milk has higher content of
A   calories.
B   water.
C   carbohydrates.
D   electrolytes.
E   iron.

2.4. Compared to human milk cow's milk contains more
A   protein.
B   phosphate.
C   vitamin K.
D   lactose.
E   sodium.

2.1. B E
Breast milk production is increased by regular and complete emptying of breast manually or a strongly sucking infant. Extra water or milk in the diet or stilboestrol do not affect breast milk production.

2.2. C D
The fat content of human milk is slightly higher than colostrum which is richer in secretory IgA and contains more protein. Colostrum has more cellular elements. Water content of the two milks is approximately the same.

2.3. D
The caloric and water content of human and cow's milk is approximately the same. The carbohydrate and iron content of human milk is greater than cow's milk. Cow's milk contains three to four times the electrolyte content of human milk.

2.4. A B C E
Compared to human milk, cow's milk contains approximately two times the amount of protein, six times the amount of phosphate, four times the amount of vitamin K and three times the amount of sodium. The lactose content of human milk is approximately twice that of cow's milk.

2.5. Which of the following formulae may be appropriate in the management of an infant with proven cow's milk protein intolerance?

A   Digestalact.
B   De-Lact.
C   Soya milk formula.
D   Pregestimil.
E   Nutramigen.

2.6. Which of the following may occur in a 2-week-old infant who has been fed on whole cow's milk?

A   An elevated blood urea nitrogen.
B   Dehydration.
C   Convulsions.
D   Elevated serum sodium.
E   Low serum calcium.

2.7. Which of the following statements regarding infant feeding is/are correct?

A   The daily fluid volume requirements per kg of pre-term babies are higher than those of full-term infants.
B   The fluid requirements of small-for-dates infants per kg are higher than those of infants who are appropriate for gestation.
C   Fat should provide 10–15% of infant's caloric intake.
D   Fully breast-fed infants do not develop infantile eczema.
E   The sugar of breast milk is the same sugar as in cow's milk.

2.8. For a full-term exclusively breastfed thriving baby, which of the following feeding practices is/are recommended?

A   Iron supplementation from the age of 2 months.
B   Fluoride supplementation of mother from delivery.
C   Vitamin C supplementation from the age of 2 months.
D   Commencement of solids at about 4 months.
E   Weaning to cow's milk at about 6 months.

2.5. C D E
In Digestalact and De-lact the lactose content of milk is changed but the milk protein is unchanged. Soya milk formula is derived from soya beans. In Pregestimil and Nutramigen the protein is hydrolysed.

2.6. A B C D E
Whole cow's milk has higher content of protein, phosphorus and electrolytes compared to human milk. As the kidney of a 2-week-old infant is unable to handle this extra load, as well as a result of metabolism of the extra protein, this results in raised blood urea nitrogen and raised serum sodium which cause osmotic diuresis resulting in dehydration. The high phosphorus prevents absorption of calcium from the gut leading to low serum calcium.

2.7. A B E
The fluid requirements of pre-term infants and small-for-dates infants are 180–200 ml/kg compared to 150 ml/kg of full-term infants who are appropriate for gestation because they have greater loss of fluid (increase of surface area relative to weight and respiratory rate). Fats provide about a third of the infant's caloric intake. Breastfeeding does not provide protection against infantile eczema. The sugar in both breast and cow's milk is lactose.

2.8. D
Full-term infants do not need iron supplementation till the age of 4–6 months as they have accumulated adequate amounts of iron in the last trimester of pregnancy. Fluoride does not appear in adequate quantities in breast milk. There is an adequate amount of vitamin C in breast milk. Solids are started at about age 4 months so that the infant is on adequate solids by the age of 6 months. Whole cow's milk can cause gastrointestinal bleeding and is not recommended till after the age of 1 year.

2.9. Which of the following statements is/are true?

A   Xerophthalmia in a 3-year-old child is pathognomonic of vitamin A deficiency.
B   Vitamin A overdose can cause raised intracranial pressure.
C   Scurvy is rare in breastfed infants.
D   Vitamin D deficiency in infants can present with seizures.
E   Vitamin E deficiency predisposes to haemolysis.

2.10. Which of the following statements concerning vitamins is/are true?

A   Mega-doses of vitamin A have been shown to be toxic.
B   Vitamin D3 (cholecalciferol) is a naturally occurring vitamin in fish oils.
C   Vitamin C is destroyed during cooking.
D   Babies fed on goat's milk require supplements of folic acid.
E   Cow's milk has less vitamin K than human milk.

2.11. Which of the following statements is/are true about vitamin C?

A   It is essential for the formation of collagen.
B   It corrects the transient tyrosinaemia in low birth weight infants.
C   Formula fed babies require vitamin C supplementation.
D   Scorbutic rosary (due to vitamin C deficiency) is indistinguishable from rachitic rosary.
E   Paucity of limb movements may be a presenting sympton of vitamin C deficiency.

2.12. Which of the following features is/are likely to be found in a 6-month-old infant with rickets?

A   Abnormal bowing of legs.
B   Convulsions.
C   Greenstick fractures.
D   Retardation of bone age.
E   Bossing of skull.

2.9. A B C D E
Xerophthalmia (dryness of conjunctiva and cornea) is due to vitamin A deficiency. Vitamin A overdose causes raised intracranial pressure. There are adequate amounts of vitamin C in breast milk. Vitamin D deficiency in infants results in hypocalcaemia and tetany as well as seizures. Vitamin E deficiency results in haemolysis due to instability of the red cell membrane.

2.10. A C D
Excess of vitamin A causes anorexia, slow growth, drying and cracking of the skin, enlargement of liver and spleen, swelling and pain of long bones, bone fragility and increased intracranial pressure. Vitamin D3 is activated 7-dehydrocholesterol which is normally present in human skin. Vitamin C is easily oxidized which is accelerated by heat, light, alkali and oxidative enzymes. Goat's milk is deficient in folic acid. Cow's milk has more vitamin K (four times) than human milk.

2.11. A B C E
Vitamin C is essential for the formation of collagen. It corrects the transient tyrosinaemia in low birth weight infants. It is destroyed during processing of milk formulae. Its deficiency results in irritability, pain in limbs due to periosteal haemorrhage which presents as pseudoparalysis. Scorbutic rosary is due to dislocation of costochondral junctions resulting in angulation which is easily distinguishable from rachitic rosary (widened epiphysis).

2.12. B C E
In rickets abnormal bowing of legs does not develop till the child begins to walk. Hypocalcaemia causes convulsions. Because of poor calcification of the bones greenstick fractures may occur. Bossing of the skull occurs because of increased formation of osteoid tissue. The bone age is not affected.

2.13. Craniotabes is significantly associated with
A   rickets.
B   osteogenesis imperfecta.
C   thalassaemia minor.
D   lacunar skull.
E   prematurity.

2.14. If the intake of calories in an infant is chronically insufficient in quantity but with a reasonable proportion derived from protein
A   he will have good subcutaneous fat stores but inadequate muscle bulk.
B   replacement of some of the carbohydrate with protein will make little difference to the clinical state of the child.
C   head growth will be markedly decreased for age.
D   weight will be decreased for age.
E   the serum protein will usually be decreased.

2.15. Biochemical abnormalities in kwashiorkor include
A   hypernatraemia.
B   aminoaciduria.
C   lactase deficiency.
D   low serum albumin.
E   potassium deficiency.

2.16. Which of the following statements is/are true of severe protein calorie malnutrition?
A   There will be normal subcutaneous fat stores but inadequate muscle bulk.
B   Replacement of some of the carbohydrate with protein will make little difference to the clinical state.
C   Total body water as percentage of body weight will be increased.
D   The serum proteins will usually be markedly decreased.
E   Total body potassium will be decreased.

2.13. A B E
In rickets and prematurity the skull is soft because of inadequate calcification. In osteogenesis imperfecta there is deficiency of bone matrix. In lacunar skull there are defects in the vault in the form of depressions or 'holes' extending to the outer surface of the skull. It occurs mainly in the frontal or parietal regions. There is no softening of the skull in thalassemia minor.

2.14. B D
In the presence of insufficient caloric intake, there is loss of subcutaneous fat tissue and weight. There is no disturbance of head growth. The serum protein will be maintained to normal values by breakdown of muscle tissue. As long as the total calories are inadequate it does not matter whether the patient eats carbohydrate or protein.

2.15. B C D E
Low serum albumin which results in oedema is the characteristic feature of kwashiorkor. Serum sodium is low or normal. Aminoaciduria results from disturbed renal function. Lactase deficiency is a result of decrease in intestinal enzymes due to subtotal villous atrophy.

2.16. B C E
In protein calorie malnutrition there is deficiency of calories which results in loss of subcutaneous fat. As the total calories remain unchanged, the protein that replaces carbohydrate will be used up to meet the caloric needs. The total body water as percentage of body weight increases as the lean body weight is proportionately increased. Unlike protein malnutrition, in protein calorie malnutrition the serum proteins are maintained because muscle tissue is being broken down to meet the caloric needs which supplies part of the protein. Total body potassium is decreased because of decrease in muscle tissue.

2.17. Failure to thrive

A   is most commonly due to an organic cause.
B   is most commonly due to lack of calories.
C   usually requires a battery of laboratory tests to determine the cause.
D   always requires documentation of caloric intake so that underfeeding due to error or ignorance is ruled out.
E   responds to feeding if the cause is organic.

2.18. A child with moderate malnutrition following a chronic diarrhoeal illness is likely to have

A   a greater fall off in length centile than of head circumference centile.
B   muscle hypotonia.
C   loss of turgor.
D   hyperkalaemia.
E   iron deficiency anaemia.

2.19. Obesity

A   is more common in infants weaned late.
B   in infancy usually leads to obesity in later life.
C   is more common in bottle-fed babies.
D   is commonly linked to adrenal gland hypersecretion.
E   is usually associated with above average height.

2.20. Which of the following is typical of an obese 8-year-old boy?

A   Greater than average height.
B   Normal bone age.
C   Normal size external genitalia.
D   Unusual happy temperament.
E   Delayed puberty.

2.17. B D
Unless obvious, organic causes of failure to thrive are uncommon. Even in developed countries the commonest cause of failure to thrive is lack of calories which is not necessarily due to inadequate availability of food, hence documentation of caloric intake is important. If the cause is organic, it will not respond to feeding alone.

2.18. A B E
In malnutrition the growth pattern that is most affected is weight followed by length and then head circumference. Muscle hypotonia results. Iron deficiency anaemia is a result of lack of absorption. Though there is low total body potassium, serum potassium is usually normal. Dehydration (loss of skin turgor) is not a prominent feature in chronic diarrhoeal illness.

2.19. B C E
Obesity is usually more common in infants that are weaned earlier. Epidemiological studies have demonstrated that obese infants grow up to be obese adults. Bottle-fed babies tend to be overfed as mothers like the bottle to be completely emptied (whether the infant wishes to finish the feed or not) which results in overfeeding. Hormonal hypersecretion is an uncommon cause of obesity. Obesity accelerates growth of height.

2.20. A C
Obesity tends to be associated with accelerated growth (including height, bone age and puberty). The external genitalia, though normal, appear to be small because of the excess amount of fat in the pubic region. The temperament is no different from other children of their age, though they may be depressed because of teasing.

2.21. Which of the following statements is/are true about juvenile obesity?

A   Inactivity of children plays a causal role.
B   The child of an obese parent has an increased chance of being obese.
C   There is some degree of insulin resistance.
D   It is associated with greater than average height.
E   In Australian urban society there is a higher incidence in lower than middle and upper economic class persons.

2.22. A 2-year-old girl is brought to see you with the complaint that she eats 'nothing'. The child is active and appears well. She weighs 11.5 kg (50th percentile) and her height is 90 cm (75th percentile). Physical examination reveals no abnormality. Which of the following statements is/are correct with regard to the management of this child?

A   She should be given a tonic.
B   She should be forced to eat.
C   She shoud be investigated for urinary tract problems.
D   Parents should be reassured that there is nothing wrong with her.
E   Parents should stop fussing about her eating.

39

2.21. A B D E
Obese children tend to be inactive which further aggravates the problem. Epidemiological studies have shown there is an increased familial incidence and a higher incidence in lower than middle or upper socio-economic classes in Australia. Obesity tends to increase height velocity. There is no evidence that there is any insulin resistance in obesity.

2.22. D E
The height and weight of this child suggest that she is growing normally. Therefore she does not need any investigations or treatment. Parents need reassurance and advised not to fuss.

3 Genetics and metabolic disorders

3.1. Concerning spontaneous early abortions (first trimester), which of the following statements is/are true?

A   The incidence of chromosome abnormalities in the abortuses is between 5 and 15%.

B   Trisomy 21 is the most frequent single chromosome abnormality in the abortuses.

C   The incidence of 45X karyotype in the abortuses is approximately the same as in the liveborn population.

D   There is an increased incidence of chromosome abnormality in parents who have had frequent (more than four) spontaneous early abortions.

E   Trisomy in an abortus implies an increased risk for trisomy in subsequent liveborn offspring.

3.2. Which of the following have been shown to be associated with an increased risk of congenital malformations?

A   Maternal pre-eclampsia.

B   Maternal diabetes.

C   Maternal ingestion of alcohol.

D   Maternal ingestion of phenytoin.

E   Maternal ingestion of salicylates.

3.3. Which of the following statements is/are true of congenital anomalies?

A   The incidence of major defects is less than 1% of total births.

B   There is an increased incidence in infants of diabetic mothers.

C   There is a recognized association between maternal oestrogen administration and infant vaginal carcinoma.

D   There is a recognized association between maternal alcoholism and cardiovascular anomalies in the infant.

E   There is a recognized association between maternal epilepsy and cleft-lip in the infant.

3.4. Which of the following can be diagnosed before 20 weeks' gestation?

A   Renal agenesis.

B   Trisomy 18 (Edwards' syndrome).

C   Beta-thalassaemia.

D   Phenylketonuria.

E   Cystic fibrosis.

3.1. D E
Routine investigations of spontaneous abortions in the first trimester have shown that at least 50% of them have chromosome abnormalities and loss of an X chromosome is the most frequent. The incidence of chromosome abnormalities in a woman increases with the increase in the number of spontaneous abortions. Trisomy in an abortus increases the risk for trisomy in subsequent liveborn offspring.

3.2. B C D
Maternal diabetes increases the risk of congenital heart disease and spinal cord malformations, maternal ingestion of alcohol increases the risk of microcephaly and facial hypoplasia and maternal ingestion of phenytoin increases the risk of facial dysplasia. There is no definite proof that maternal ingestion of salicylates causes any congenital malformations though premature closure of ductus arteriosus has been implicated. Maternal pre-eclampsia unless associated with some other problems is not a recognized cause of congenital malformation.

3.3. B C E
The incidence of major congenital malformations is about 1% of total births. It is increased in infants of diabetic mothers. Oestrogen administration to pregnant women has been demonstrated to increase the incidence of vaginal carcinoma in their infants. Although maternal alcoholism can cause microcephaly, facial hypoplasia and disturbance of growth, cardiovascular anomalies are not associated with it. The infants of mothers with epilepsy have a high incidence of cleft lip but it is not clear whether this is due to the anticonvulsants or the underlying disease process.

3.4. A B C E
Before 20 weeks, renal agenesis can be diagnosed by ultrasound, trisomy by chromosome cultures (fibroblast from amniotic fluid) and beta-thalassaemia by fetal blood sampling. Cystic fibrosis can be diagnosed by DNA analysis of a chorionic villus biopsy if an index case is known. There is no test available for prenatal diagnosis of phenylketonuria.

3.5. Antenatal diagnosis is available for which of the following?
A   Down's syndrome.
B   Neurofibromatosis.
C   Congenital adrenal hyperplasia.
D   Myelomeningocele.
E   Diabetes mellitus.

3.6. Which of the following is/are true of autosomal dominant diseases?
A   They are manifest in heterozygotes for the relevant defective gene.
B   They typically affect multiple members of only one sibship in a family.
C   The probability of being affected, for the relative of an affected person, is influenced by the penetrance.
D   A parent of an affected person must be heterozygous.
E   They are usually lethal.

3.7. Which of the following conditions have an autosomal dominant inheritance?
A   Cystic fibrosis.
B   Thalassaemia major.
C   Achondroplasia.
D   Neurofibromatosis.
E   Phenylketonuria.

3.8. In a disease such as achondroplasia where the inheritance is invariably autosomal dominant with complete penetrance, which of the following is/are true?
A   The risk of achondroplasia to each offspring of an affected person is 50%.
B   The risk to the sibling of an affected person who has normal parents is 50%.
C   There is an increased frequency of consanguinity in the parents of affected people.
D   All the offspring of two achondroplastic parents will be affected.
E   The abnormal gene is on the X chromosome.

3.5. A C D
Antenatal diagnosis of Down's syndrome can be made by amniotic fluid examination and culture of the fibroblasts, congenital adrenal hyperplasia by demonstrating raised levels of 17-hydroxyprogesterone and delta-4 androstenedione in the amniotic fluid, myelomeningocele by demonstrating raised levels of alpha-fetoprotein in the amniotic fluid or by ultrasound. There is no antenatal technique available for diagnosis of neurofibromatosis and diabetes mellitus.

3.6. A C
Autosomal dominant diseases will manifest if the defective gene is present in heterozygotes. Most autosomal dominant diseases are due to fresh mutations and therefore they do not affect multiple members of one sibship or may not be present in the parent. The majority of autosomal dominant diseases are not lethal and the incidence in relatives of affected persons is influenced by the penetrance – there may be skipping of a generation.

3.7. C D
Achondroplasia and neurofibromatosis are autosomal dominant diseases. Cystic fibrosis, thalassaemia major and phenylketonuria are inherited recessively.

3.8. A
Achondroplasia is autosomal dominant (80% are fresh mutants). The risk to the offspring of an affected person will be 50%. Consanguinity does not increase the risk in offspring unless both parents are achondroplastic. If both parents are achondroplastic, 25% of the children wil be normal. The exact position of the gene on the chromosome has not been identified.

3.9. A young couple have learnt that the wife's father, aged 42 years, has Huntington's disease (Huntington's chorea). They have a son and a daughter. Which of the following statements is/are true?

A On the above information alone, each of their children has 1 chance in 4 of being affected.

B If the wife is still unaffected at the age of 50 years, her offspring will no longer be at risk.

C The chromosome bearing the defective gene has been identified.

D Huntington's disease is sex-linked dominant.

E Huntington's disease is due to a new mutation gene in a high proportion of cases.

3.10. Which of the following is/are true of autosomal recessive diseases?

A Parental consanguinity increases the risk to offspring.

B Skipping of generations is characteristic.

C Each future sibling of an affected child has one chance in four in being similarly affected.

D For parents of an affected child, artificial insemination from an unrelated donor is a genetically sound option.

E They are symptomatically manifest in persons heterozygous for the defective genes.

3.11. The incidence of a disease within the population of an autosomal recessive condition is approximately 1 in 2500. Which of the following statements is/are correct?

A The frequency of the heterozygote state is 1 in 250.

B The frequency of the heterozygote state is 1 in 25.

C The chance of two carriers of this condition having an affected child is 50%.

D The chance of the disease occurring in each child born to parents both of whom are carriers, is 25%.

E If this condition is lethal at birth, ⅔ of the siblings will be heterozygous.

3.12. Which of the following is/are inherited as an autosomal recessive condition?

A Phenylketonuria.

B Cystic fibrosis.

C Factor VIII deficiency (haemophilia).

D Neurofibromatosis.

E Congenital adrenal hyperplasia.

3.9. A C
Huntington's chorea is an autosomal dominant disease and therefore the daughter (wife) has a 50% chance of having the disease, as a result her children have a 25% chance of being affected. The disease may present at any age though it usually manifests after the age of 40 years. The defective gene has been identified to be on chromosome 4. It is not sex-linked and mutations are uncommon.

3.10. A C D
All individuals have a number of abnormal recessive genes. The chance of two individuals having the same abnormal recessive genes are increased in close relatives and therefore parental consanguinity would increase the risk of recessive diseases in offspring. Each future sibling of an affected child has a 25% chance of being similarly affected ($\frac{1}{2} \times \frac{1}{2}$). Unless the donor also has a recessive gene (which is usually rare), artificial insemination from an unrelated donor is likely to result in a normal offspring. Autosomal recessive diseases do not manifest in heterozygous persons because the 'normal dominant' gene does not allow the recessive gene to manifest. There is no skipping of generations.

3.11. B D E
The gene frequency of an autosomal recessive disease is calculated by the formula $4 \times X^2$ where X is the frequency. In the problem presented it will be 1 in 25. In autosomal recessive diseases the chance of two parents having an affected child ($\frac{1}{2} \times \frac{1}{2}$) and a normal child ($\frac{1}{2} \times \frac{1}{2}$) is 25%. The other two children would be heterozygous. If the condition is lethal at birth, $\frac{2}{3}$ of the siblings will be heterozygous.

3.12. A B E
Phenylketonuria, cystic fibrosis and congenital adrenal hyperplasia are autosomal recessive diseases. Factor VIII deficiency is X-linked recessive. Neurofibromatosis is autosomal dominant.

3.13. Amanda and Alan are first cousins. They seek genetic advice. They are in normal health. Which of the following statements is/are true?

A The average incidence of birth defects in their offspring is closer to 1 in 20 than to 1 in 4.

B The risk for birth defects in their offspring would be greater if their parents were also first cousins.

C Their offspring are at increased risk for autosomal dominant disorders.

D Their offspring are at increased risk for autosomal recessive disorders.

E Their sons are at increased risk for sex-linked recessive disorders.

3.14. A 38-year-old woman has an only son in whom haemophilia is diagnosed. Her brother is also affected. Which of the following statements is/are correct?

A The condition is X-linked dominant.

B All her future daughters will be carriers.

C All of her son's daughters will be carriers.

D Her son's sons will be at 50% risk of haemophilia.

E Fetal diagnosis of haemophilia for future pregnancy by DNA analysis is possible.

3.15. Bertha has a brother and a maternal uncle with haemophilia A. Her sister has a mild but significant bleeding tendency. Which of the following statements is/are true?

A The risk of haemophilia in Bertha's first offspring, if male, is 1 in 4.

B The bleeding tendency in Bertha's sister indicates that the defective gene is autosomal in this family.

C Bertha's mother is an obligate carrier.

D Prenatal diagnosis of haemophlia A has been achieved.

E If Bertha had unaffected sons, this would influence the probability that she is a carrier.

3.16. Which of the following statements is/are true of a recessive disorder carried on the X chromosome?

A It cannot be passed from a man to his son.

B It can affect males.

C It will usually not affect females.

D The gene will be carried by all the daughters of an affected man.

E It is the commonest form of sex-linked inheritance.

3.13. A D

First cousins are likely to have many recessive genes common to both of them. They are also likely to have other genes in common. Therefore their children are at greater risk of having autosomal recessive disorders. However, the risk of having birth defects due to multifactoral causes are greater than those due to recessive disorders. The risk of autosomal dominant disorders and sex-linked recessive disorders is not affected. The risk of birth defects in the offsprings of first cousin marriages is no greater even if their parents were first cousins.

3.14. C

Haemophilia is X-linked recessive. 50% of the daughters of a carrier will be carriers and all the daughters of an affected son will be carriers and her son's sons will not be affected. Antenatal diagnosis by DNA analysis is not possible.

3.15. A C D E

Haemophilia is sex-linked recessive. The chances of Bertha being a carrier is 1 in 2 and therefore the chances of having a male child with haemophilia is 1 in 4 for every male child. The family tree shows strongly that the disease is X-linked recessive and Bertha's mother is a carrier. Prenatal diagnosis of haemophilia A can be made by examination of the fetal blood. With each unaffected son, the probability that Bertha is not a carrier is increased.

3.16. A B C D E

X-linked recessive disorders are passed on to all the daughters of an affected man. The daughters are carriers and do not manifest the disease but pass on to half of their sons. X-linked recessive disorders are the most common form of sex-linked inheritance.

3.17. Which of the following are determined by monogenic (simple Mendelian) inheritance?
A   Congenital adrenocortical hyperplasia.
B   Galactosaemia.
C   Spina bifida.
D   Down's syndrome.
E   Cystic fibrosis of the pancreas.

3.18. Which of the following conditions may have polygenic inheritance?
A   Galactosaemia.
B   Talipes.
C   Meningomyelocele.
D   Polydactyly.
E   Turner's syndrome.

3.19. Which of the following is/are true of the clinical features of Down's syndrome?
A   Translocation Down's syndrome is clinically less severe than trisomic Down's syndrome.
B   Congenital heart disease is present in more than 70% of cases.
C   Mosaic Down's syndrome is compatible with normal intelligence.
D   Most non-mosaic cases function intellectually in the mildly handicapped range.
E   The incidence of hypothyroidism is greater than in the general population.

3.20. Which of the following statements is/are true of Down's syndrome?
A   All cases are due to trisomy 21 (47 XX or XY, + 21).
B   In more than 90% of cases, parents' chromosomes are normal.
C   Examination of the parents' chromosomes may alter the assessment of recurrence risk in sibs.
D   The mortality rate in utero exceeds 25%.
E   Incidence at birth, at maternal age 40–45 is more than twice that at maternal age 20–25.

3.17. A B E
Congenital adrenocortical hyperplasia, galactosaemia and cystic fibrosis are single genes recessive conditions. The inheritance of spina bifida is multifactorial. Down's syndrome is a chromosomal disorder.

3.18. B C
Talipes and meningomyelocele are due to polygenic inheritance. Galactosaemia is recessive, polydactyly is autosomal dominant and Turner's syndrome is due to a chromosome abnormality (XO). Some cases of talipes are due to abnormal posture in utero.

3.19. C E
There is no relationship to the severity of the manifestation of Down's syndrome whether it is translocation or trisomy. Congenital heart disease is present in about 40% of cases. Children with mosaic Down's syndrome can have normal intelligence. Non-mosaic cases are moderately retarded. The incidence of hypothyroidism is increased.

3.20. B C D E
Down's syndrome may be due to trisomy 21 (95%) or due to 15/21 translocation. More than 50% of trisomy 21 fetuses are spontaneously aborted during early pregnancy. The incidence in the general population is 1 in 600–800 compared to 5% in mothers over the age of 40 years. Examination of the parents' chromosomes helps to identify parents who have a balanced 15/21 chromosome and as such will help in the assessment of recurrence risk in siblings. Other than those parents who have balanced translocation (less than 10%), the chromosomes are normal in both parents.

3.21. Which of the following eye signs is/are likely to be found in infants with Down's syndrome?
A   Epicanthic folds.
B   Bitot spots.
C   Congenital glaucoma.
D   Brushfield spots.
E   Oblique palpebral fissures.

3.22. A child with Down's syndrome has an increased risk of
A   hydrocephalus.
B   acyanotic congenital heart disease.
C   duodenal atresia.
D   leukaemia.
E   refractive error.

3.23. Which of the following statements is/are true of individuals with chromosome constitution 45 XO (sometimes written 45 X)?
A   They are phenotypically male.
B   They are phenotypically female, with male hair distribution developing during adolescence.
C   They are of short stature.
D   Hormone treatment is appropriate.
E   There is an increased incidence of systemic hypertension.

3.24. Which of the following is/are recognized features of XO-Turner syndrome?
A   Aortic abnormalities.
B   Infertility.
C   Short stocky build with shield-like chest.
D   Pigmented naevi.
E   Lymphoedema.

3.21. A D E
The eye signs of Down's syndrome include oblique palpebral fissures, epicanthic folds, speckled iris (Brushfield spots) and cataracts. Bitot spots are due to vitamin A deficiency. Congenital glaucoma is not a feature of Down's syndrome.

3.22. B C D E
Children with Down's syndrome have congenital heart disease (mainly septal defect) especially of the endocardial cushion which does not present with cyanosis. Gastrointestinal manifestations include duodenal atresia and Hirschsprung's disease. They have an increased incidence of refractive errors and of leukaemia which is of the lymphatic type.

3.23. C D E
Individuals with karyotype 45XO are phenotypically female with hair distribution similar to females at adolescence. About 15% of patients have coarctation of aorta and can present with hypertension which may also be found in a few patients without known aetiology. Majority of patients need oestrogen replacement therapy at puberty.

3.24. A B C D E
Aortic abnormalities in XO-Turner syndrome include coarctation and dissecting aneurysm. Infertility is due to gonadal dysgenesis. They have a broad chest which gives an illusion of widely spaced nipples. Pigmented naevi appear with increasing age. Other features include lymphoedema, webbing of neck, cutibus valgus and hyperconvex fingernails.

3.25. Monozygotic twins have
A   a shared placental circulation.
B   more frequent concordance for congenital malformation than dizygotic twins.
C   placenta and membranes from which diagnosis of monozygosity can be made readily.
D   a greater frequency than dizygotic twins.
E   increased familial incidence.

3.26. A specific enzyme defect has been demonstrated in
A   Down's syndrome.
B   hypoglycaemia in small-for-date infants.
C   hereditary spherocytosis.
D   phenylketonuria.
E   methylmalonic aciduria.

3.27. Which of the following substances give(s) a positive test for reducing substances in urine?
A   Galactose.
B   Sucrose.
C   Fructose.
D   Lactose.
E   Phenylpyruvic acid.

3.28. Presence of reducing substances in urine is suggestive of which of the following disorders?
A   Coeliac disease.
B   Galactosaemia.
C   Cystic fibrosis.
D   Diabetes mellitus.
E   Phenylketonuria.

3.25. A B

The vascular anastomosis in monozygotic twins may be artery to artery or vein to vein or artery to vein. Monozygotic twins show a more frequent concordance for congenital malformations than dizygotic twins. It is not possible with 100% certainty to establish monozygosity by examination of the placenta and membranes. However, the diagnosis of dizygosity can be made with more certainty. The incidence of monozygotic twins is less than dizygotic twins. There is no familial predisposition in monozygotic twins.

3.26. D E

Phenylketonuria is caused by deficiency of phenylalanine hydroxylase. Methylmalonic aciduria is due to deficiency of methylmalonyl CoA mutase. No enzyme deficiency has been demonstrated in Down's syndrome and hereditary spherocytosis. The hypoglycaemia in the small-for-dates infant is due to low energy reserves.

3.27. A C D

Galactose, fructose and lactose are reducing substances and when present in urine will give a positive test. Sucrose and phenylpyruvic acid do not reduce sugar.

3.28. B D

In coeliac disease and phenylketonuria there are no reducing substances in the urine. In galactosaemia there is lactose in the urine and in diabetes mellitus there is glucose in the urine which are reducing substances. In cystic fibrosis usually there is no reducing substance in the urine unless the patient develops diabetes mellitus.

3.29. **Elevated plasma phenylalanine in women can cause their offspring to have**
A   reduction deformities of limbs.
B   clinical phenylketonuria.
C   mental retardation.
D   persistent hyperphenylalaninaemia.
E   transient hyperphenylalaninaemia.

3.30. In which of the following may glucose appear in the urine?
A   Fanconi syndrome.
B   Congenital adrenal hyperplasia.
C   Cerebral haemorrhage.
D   Galactosaemia.
E   Salicylate intoxication.

3.29. C E
Elevated plasma phenylalanine levels in pregnant women can result in elevated plasma phenylalanine levels in their fetuses which will cause mental retardation. The blood will show a raised phenylalanine level a few days after birth but will return to normal if the infant does not have true phenylketonuria. Classical phenylketonuria will not result unless the father is a carrier or has phenylketonuria. Phenylketonuria in women does not cause any deformity of the limbs in their offspring.

3.30. A C E
In Fanconi syndrome there is glycosuria and aminoaciduria, in cerebral haemorrhage and salicylate intoxication there is hyperglycaemia which results in glucose being present in the urine. In galactosaemia there is lactose in the urine which may be confused with glucose because both are reducing substances. In salicylate poisoning there is hyperglycaemia and glycosuria.

4   Fetal and neonatal medicine

4.1. Routine newborn screening on filter paper blood spot is possible for which of the following conditions?
A   Thalassaemia major.
B   Hypothyroidism.
C   G-6-PD deficiency.
D   Cystic fibrosis.
E   Galactosemia.

4.2. Which of the following statements is/are true of a normal full-term infant on the first day of life?
A   Fluid requirements are 100 ml/kg on the first day.
B   The average head circumference is 29 cm.
C   The urinary output is 1–3 ml/kg.
D   A true blood glucose of 2 mmol/l is within the normal range.
E   The average blood pressure is 50–60 mmHg.

4.3. Which of the following may resolve spontaneously?
A   Eosinophilic rash (erythema toxicum).
B   Port-wine stains.
C   Capillary haemangioma.
D   Cephalhaematoma.
E   Vaginal tag.

4.4 Which of the following statements concerning newborn babies is/are correct?
A   Jaundice occurring on the first day of life is pathological.
B   Hydrocele should be drained as early as possible to avoid testicular atrophy.
C   Eosinophilic rash (erythema toxicum) is an allergic manifestation.
D   Ductus arteriousus usually closes physiologically within 48 hours.
E   Facial petechiae at birth are indicative of haemorrhagic disease.

4.1.   B D E
Screening for hypothyroidism, cystic fibrosis and galactosaemia is carried out by measuring TSH, immunoreactive trypsin and galactose-1-phosphate in the blood spot.

4.2.   C D E
The fluid requirements of a full-term infant on the first day of life are 60 ml/kg, the average head circumference is 35 cm and urinary output is 1–3 ml/kg. The blood sugar range is 1.5–4 mmol/l. The average blood pressure is 50–60 mmHg.

4.3.   A C D E
Erythema toxicum is a rash of unknown aetiology which waxes and wanes, capillary haemangiomas may grow faster than the baby initially but resolve eventually. Cephalhaematomas usually resolve within 6–12 weeks and vaginal tags drop off spontaneously. Port-wine stains are permanent but they may appear less prominent as they do not grow at the same rate as the infant.

4.4.   A D
Jaundice appearing on the first day of life is usually haemolytic or due to intrauterine infection. Most hydroceles in the neonatal period resolve spontaneously. The aetiology of eosinophilic rash is not known. Physiological closure of the ductus arteriosus occurs within few hours of birth due to high oxygen tension in the aorta. Facial petechiae can occur in any condition which causes obstruction of flow of blood from the head and neck.

4.5. Which of the following statements is/are correct?

A   Gestational age of 35 weeks + 6 days should be considered as 36 weeks.
B   Pre-term infant is defined as a baby with gestation of less than 35 weeks.
C   Small-for-dates babies are more common than large-for-dates.
D   Postmature infants are more than 42 weeks' gestation.
E   Neonatal period extends up to 30 days of life.

4.6. Which of the following statements is/are correct?

A   The infant mortality rate is the number of deaths in the first year of life per 1000 live births.
B   The neonatal mortality rate is the number of deaths in the first four weeks of life per 1000 live births.
C   The neonatal mortality rate has decreased more quickly than the infant mortality rate over the last fifty years.
D   The perinatal mortality rate is the number of stillbirths plus first week deaths per 1000 total births.
E   The perinatal mortality rate is determined mainly by the effectiveness of paediatric services.

4.7. Infants born to heroin-addicted mothers

A   are unexpectedly 'large-for-dates'.
B   have a high incidence of neonatal jaundice.
C   have been conclusively shown to have a higher incidence of congenital defects.
D   in the withdrawal phase are often tachypnoeic and have a respiratory alkalosis.
E   may not manifest withdrawal symptoms until one week after birth.

4.8. A baby of 40 weeks' gestation is born weighing 2000 g. Which of the following statements is/are likely to be true of this infant?

A   He is premature.
B   He is at risk of hypoglycaemia.
C   His mother is a prediabetic.
D   He is at risk of developing meconium aspiration.
E   His head circumference is likely to be on a similar percentile to his weight.

4.5. D
Gestational age is stated as completed weeks. A pre-term infant is defined as an infant less than 37 weeks' gestation (i.e. 36 weeks, 6 days). Neonatal period is defined as the first 28 days of life. Infants who are small for date (less than 10th percentile) and large for date (more than 90th percentile) are equal in number. Postmaturity is more than 42 weeks' gestation.

4.6. A B
The infant is defined as a child between birth and 1 year, a neonate is a child between birth and 28 days and perinatal is defined as the period from 20 weeks' gestation to 28 days' postnatal life. Mortality rates are expressed per 1000 births. Infant mortality rate has decreased dramatically over the last 50 years because of improvement in child health programmes (nutrition and immunization). In contrast, conditions causing neonatal mortality (prematurity and its complications, congenital malformations) are poorly understood. As a result there has been a slower reduction in neonatal mortality rate. The greatest improvement in perinatal mortality has been as a result of improvement in obstetric services.

4.7. D E
Infants born to heroin-addicted mothers are small-for-dates, have a lower incidence of neonatal jaundice, have no congenital abnormalities and may not manifest symptoms for 1–4 weeks after birth. They have respiratory problems including tachypnoea which may result in alkalosis.

4.8. B D
This baby is a small-for-dates infant born at term and is likely to have hypoglycaemia and intrapartum asphyxia. Infants of prediabetic mothers are large-for-dates. As the head continues to grow in spite of intrauterine growth retardation the head circumference is likely to be on a higher percentile than the weight.

4.9. A 25-year-old para 1 mother gave birth to twin boys at 38 weeks' gestation. Twin A weighed 3200 g and twin B weighed 2400 g at birth. Which of the following statements is/are correct?

A   The weight of twin B is appropriate for gestational age and twin A is large for gestational age.
B   The weight of twin A is appropriate for gestational age and twin B is small for gestational age.
C   Neither infant is appropriate weight for twins at 38 weeks' gestation.
D   Both infants are large for twins at 38 weeks' gestation.
E   There is an increased risk in twin B of hypoglycaemia.

4.10. Which of the following have more than a chance association with the small-for-dates infant?

A   A high perinatal mortality.
B   Congenital malformation.
C   Permanent physical or mental retardation.
D   Idiopathic respiratory distress syndrome (hyaline membrane disease).
E   High haematocrit.

4.11. Which of the following neonatal problems is/are seen more frequently in the infant of diabetic mothers?

A   Hypoglycaemia.
B   Hyaline membrane disease.
C   Polycythaemia.
D   Hyperbilirubinaemia.
E   Congenital malformations.

4.12. Which of the following conditions is polyhydramnios a recognized complication of pregnancy?

A   Anencephaly.
B   Oesophageal atresia.
C   Maternal diabetes mellitus.
D   Renal agenesis.
E   Ileal atresia.

4.9. B E
The average weight at term is 3.3–3.5 kg. A weight of 2.4 kg is below the 10th percentile. Twin B is likely to develop hypoglycaemia because of being small-for-dates.

4.10. A B C E
Small-for-dates infants have intrauterine stress which results in increased perinatal morbidity, mortality and high haematocrit. Permanent physical or mental retardation may occur if the aetiology is intrauterine infection or chromosomal abnormality. There is a strong association between congenital malformations and small-for-dates infants. Idiopathic respiratory distress syndrome is less likely to occur because intrauterine stress results in maturation of lung.

4.11. A B C D E
Infants of diabetic mothers will develop hypoglycaemia (because of increased production of insulin by the infant's pancreas) and hyaline membrane disease especially if the diabetes is poorly controlled. These infants have polycythaemia and are likely to develop hyperbilirubinaemia. Infants of diabetic mothers tend to have neurological malformations (hydrocephalus, spina bifida, sacral agenesis) and congential heart disease.

4.12. A B C
Polyhydramnios may occur in association with any major congenital malformation but particularly with anencephaly. It is a recognized association of maternal diabetes. Oesophageal atresia causes polyhydramnios because the fetus is unable to swallow the amniotic fluid. In renal agenesis there is oligohydramnios. Midgut and colonic atresias do not affect the volume of liquor amnii.

4.13. Central nervous system abnormalities associated with the fetal alcohol syndrome include
A   mild to moderate mental retardation.
B   microcephaly.
C   irritability in the neonatal period.
D   hyperactivity in childhood.
E   macroscopic changes in the brain.

4.14. Which of the following statements is/are true of alpha-fetoprotein (AFP)?
A   Its concentration in amniotic fluid is increased in fetal intestinal atresia.
B   In amniotic fluid its concentration is maximum at 12–14 weeks' gestation.
C   In maternal serum its maximum concentration is at 26 weeks' gestation.
D   Main site of synthesis of AFP is the fetal spinal cord.
E   AFP levels are normal in closed meningoceles.

4.15. Which of the following statements is/are true of second trimester prenatal diagnosis?
A   Diagnosis of neural tube defect requires cultivation of amniocytes.
B   It is possible to diagnose polycystic disease of kidneys.
C   The risk of fetal death (i.e. unintended abortion) associated with amniocentesis is about 5% in experienced hands.
D   DNA for diagnostic testing may be obtained from amniotic fluid.
E   Examination of maternal blood may lead to diagnosis of neural tube defect.

4.16. Which of the following conditions is/are recognized to be associated with respiratory difficulties in newborn infants?
A   Funnel chest (pectus excavatum).
B   Oesophageal atresia.
C   Oligohydramnios.
D   Bilateral choanal atresia.
E   Micrognathia (receding chin) with cleft palate.

4.13. A B C D E
Alcohol causes alterations in growth and morphogenesis which will result in mental retardation, microcephaly, irritability in the neonatal period, hyperactivity in childhood and macroscopic changes in the brain.

4.14. A E
In amniotic fluid alpha-fetoprotein is maximum between 14–18 weeks of gestation. Serum concentrations are highest between 16–18 weeks of gestation. It is synthesized by the fetal liver. Levels are raised in anencephaly and open meningomyeloceles but not in closed meningoceles. Its amniotic fluid concentration is also increased by the presence of fetal blood, fetal abortion or death, Rh disease, congenital nephrosis, omphalocele, intestinal atresia and Meckel's syndrome.

4.15. B D E
Diagnosis of neural tube defect is made by examination of alphafetoprotein or by ultrasound. The size of the kidneys can be clearly defined during the second trimester of pregnancy. The risk of abortion following amniocentesis is about 1%. DNA may be obtained from the amniotic cells in the amniotic fluid for diagnosis. Maternal serum alphafetoprotein will be high at 18 weeks' gestation with open neural tube defects.

4.16. B C D E
Funnel chest causes no respiratory symptoms. The respiratory difficulties in oesophageal atresia are due to aspiration of secretions into the lung, in oligohydramnios are due to lung hypoplasia, in bilateral choanal atresia because newborn infants are obligate nose breathers in micrognathia with cleft palate (Pierre–Robin syndrome) due to obstruction of breathing by the falling back of the tongue.

4.17. Major function(s) of surfactant is/are to
A increase the tendency of the lungs to collapse.
B increase pulmonary compliance.
C lubricate the alveoli.
D decrease alveolar surface tension.
E decrease the work of breathing.

4.18. Diaphragmatic hernia in the newborn
A is more common on the right side than the left.
B is associated with pulmonary hypoplasia.
C may be asymptomatic.
D characteristically causes vomiting.
E has more than a chance association with malrotation of the gut.

4.19. An infant is delivered at 32 weeks' gestation. He develops respiratory distress soon after birth with marked chest recession. At the age of 4 hours he has a cyanotic episode. Chest X-ray shows ground-glass appearance with an air bronchogram. This presentation is consistent with the diagnosis of
A hyaline membrane disease.
B meconium aspiration.
C wet lung.
D bacterial infection.
E tracheo-oesophageal fistula.

4.20. Which of the following statements is/are true in newborn infants?
A The most useful indicator of response to resuscitation is heart rate.
B A low 1-minute Apgar score correlates well with long-term prognosis.
C Hypoxia is more likely to cause brain damage in pre-term babies than in full-term babies.
D A normal cord blood IgM excludes a congenital viral infection.
E Convulsions following hypoxia in full-term infants indicate a poor prognosis.

4.17. D E
Surfactant lowers alveolar surface tension which maintains alveolar stability and decreases lung compliance and work of breathing.

4.18. B C E
Diaphragmatic hernia is more common on the left, is associated with pulmonary hypoplasia because of the gut contents in the thorax and does not cause vomiting. There is often incomplete rotation of the gut. Some patients may be diagnosed on routine chest X-ray.

4.19. A D
Prematurity, respiratory distress syndrome and the X-ray appearances described are consistent with hyaline membrane disease which is indistinguishable from bacterial infection. The X-ray appearances are not consistent with meconium aspiration, wet lung and tracheo-oesophageal fistula.

4.20. A E
Heart rate rises in severely asphyxiated infants following resuscitation before sustained spontaneous respiration is established. The 1-minute Apgar score does not correlate well with long-term prognosis. A better indicator of long-term prognosis is the 5-minute Apgar score. Brain damage occurs more readily in the mature brain. While raised cord blood IgM occurs in congenital viral infections, it is not always present in all cases. Convulsions following hypoxia are usually due to hypoxic ischaemic encephalopathy and indicate a poor prognosis.

4.21. Perinatal asphyxia has been implicated in the causation of
A   necrotizing enterocolitis.
B   meconium inhalation.
C   hypoglycaemia.
D   renal failure.
E   intraventricular haemorrhage.

4.22. A newborn has an asymmetrical Moro reflex. The grasp reflex is preserved for the affected arm which is weak. There is limitation in abduction and external rotation movements of the shoulder and supination of the forearm. The neurological lesion involves
A   motor cortex on contralateral side.
B   third and fourth cervical nerves.
C   fifth and sixth cervical nerves.
D   seventh and eighth cervical nerves.
E   first and second thoracic nerves.

4.23. Which of the following statements is/are true of an infant with severe asphyxia neonatorum (cord blood pH 6.9) who has no further respiratory problems?
A   Blood pH will be more than 7.35 at the age of 4 hours.
B   There will be a decrease in urinary output in the first 48 hours.
C   Examination of urine will show haematuria and proteinuria in more than 50% of cases.
D PCO_2 will probably be below normal at the age of 8 hours.
E   Administration of dexamethasone will not affect outcome.

4.24. Which of the following statements is/are true?
A   Jaundice appearing at 12 hours after birth would suggest a greatly impaired glucuronyl transferase activity.
B   During fetal life products of fetal haemoglobin breakdown are cleared by passage into the amniotic fluid.
C   There is no risk of kernicterus in biliary atresia.
D   Biliary atresia is readily distinguished from neonatal hepatitis by liver function test.
E   In newborn infants, beta-thalassaemia increases risk of hyperbilirubin-aemia.

4.21. A B C D E
Perinatal asphyxia causes necrotizing enterocolitis as a result of ischaemia of gut, passage of meconium into the liquor leading to inhalation, hypoglycaemia due to anaerobic metabolism of glycogen, renal failure due to renal tubular necrosis and intraventricular haemorrhage due to cerebral ischaemia and disturbances of cerebral blood flow.

4.22. C
The muscles innervated by the fifth and sixth cervical roots are deltoid, biceps, brachioradialis and supinator, which are some of the movements affected described in the stem.

4.23. B C D E
The patient would have suffered severe metabolic acidosis and therefore blood pH would not return to normal till the age of 24–48 hours. Urine output is decreased because of damage to the renal tubules (due to hypoxia) which is manifested as haematuria and proteinuria. The PCO_2 would be low because of hyperventilation due to metabolic acidosis. Dexamethasone has not been demonstrated to affect the outcome.

4.24. C
Jaundice appearing in the first 24 hours is usually due to haemolysis. Most of fetal haemoglobin breakdown products are cleared via the placenta. In biliary atresia there is conjugated hyperbilirubinaemia which does not cause kernicterus. The results of liver function test (enzymes, alkaline phosphatase) may be similar in both neonatal hepatitis and biliary atresia. There is no increased risk of hyperbilirubinaemia due to beta-thalassaemia as newborn infants normally have haemoglobin F.

4.25. Which of the following statements is/are true of physiological jaundice?

A It rarely (<5%) presents before the age of 24 hours.
B It is due mainly to temporarily impaired hepatic clearance of bilirubin.
C In premature infants it may persist for 3–4 weeks.
D Direct bilirubin levels may be as high as indirect bilirubin levels.
E It may cause kernicterus.

4.26. Which of the following conditions have more than a chance association with non-conjugated hyperbilirubinaemia in the first month of life?

A Hypothyroidism.
B Breast feeding.
C Biliary atresia.
D Beta-thalassaemia major.
E Intestinal obstruction.

4.27. Which of the following cause conjugated hyperbilirubinaemia persisting beyond 14 days of life?

A Breast-milk jaundice.
B Galactosaemia.
C Congenital hypothyroidism.
D Biliary atresia.
E Congenital syphilis.

4.28. The radiological findings in advanced cases of necrotizing enterocolitis of infancy characteristically include

A pneumatosis intestinalis.
B gas in portal vein.
C free gas in the peritonal cavity.
D colonic spasm.
E bubbly granular appearance.

4.25. A B C
Physiological jaundice rarely appears before the age of 24–48 hours and is due mainly to hepatic immaturity. It persists longer in premature infants. Direct bilirubin levels are less than 10% of the total bilirubin. Levels are never high enough to cause kernicterus.

4.26. A B E
Unconjugated hyperbilirubinaemia persists in hypothyroidism due to slow metabolism. In breastfeeding and intestinal obstruction there is an increased load of bilirubin from the enterohepatic circulation. As the haemoglobin of a normal full-term newborn infant is about 70% HbF there is no increase in bilirubin load in beta-thalassaemia major in the newborn.

4.27. B D E
The direct hyperbilirubinaemia in galactosaemia and congenital syphilis is due to destruction of liver architecture. In biliary atresia it is due to obstruction of flow of the bile. Breast-milk jaundice and congenital hypothyroidism cause unconjugated hyperbilirubinaemia.

4.28. A B C
Pneumatosis intestinalis and gas in portal vein are due to the presence of gas-producing organisms in the bowel wall. The free gas in the peritoneum indicates perforation. Colonic spasm is not a feature of necrotizing enterocolitis. Bubbly granular appearance is seen in meconium ileus.

4.29. Which of the following statements is/are correct?

A A platelet count of 50 000/cmm is normal in a full-term infant aged 12 hours.

B There is an increase in haemoglobin level within 3 hours of birth.

C The gradual fall in haemoglobin in the first 2 weeks of life is due to instability of fetal haemoglobin.

D Anaemia in a premature infant aged 4 weeks is most likely due to poor iron store.

E Blood loss is the commonest cause of non-haemolytic anaemia in the newborn.

4.30. A 32-year-old gravida 2, para 1, group O Rh-negative woman delivers her second child at 38 weeks' gestation. During her pregnancy her Rh antibodies titre rose from 1:8 to 1:32. The cord blood examination shows blood group A Rh-positive, Coombs' test negative, serum bilirubin 35 μmol/l. Which of the following statements is/are correct?

A The baby does not have Rh-isoimmunization.

B The mother should be given anti-D gammaglobulin within three days of delivery.

C The baby is at great risk to develop hyperbilirubinaemia requiring phototherapy.

D The rise in antibody titre during the pregnancy was unrelated to the baby's Rh status.

E The mother should have had amniocentesis during her pregnancy.

4.31. In a full-term infant weighing 3.5 kg

A digestive tract lacks some of the enzymes needed for digestion of milk products.

B supplemental iron therapy is indicated from the age of 3 weeks.

C subconjunctival haemorrhage is most likely to be due to strangulation by cord around the neck.

D erythema toxicum indicates skin allergy.

E blood volume is about 300 ml.

4.32. Which of the following statements is/are true of an infant born with erythroblastosis due to Rh isoimmunization?

A His mother should be given 1 ml of anti-D gammaglobulin within 72 hours of delivery.

B Acidosis will increase the risk of kernicterus in the presence of hyper-bilirubinaemia.

C If an exchange transfusion is required it is desirable to use blood of the mother's Rh group.

D His mother will have a positive direct Coombs' test.

E Anaemia may become increasingly a problem after the jaundice has subsided.

4.29. B E
The platelet count in a full-term infant is between 150 000 and 250 000. The increase in haemoglobin level soon after birth is due to moving of the fluid from the vascular to the extravascular compartment. The gradual fall of haemoglobin in the first 2 weeks of life is mainly due to 'physiological hypoplasia' of marrow. Anaemia in the premature infant at 4 weeks is most likely due to frequent blood sampling or due to rapid growth. Blood loss (usually occurs at birth which may be obvious or may occur into the maternal circulation) is the commonest cause of non-haemolytic anaemia in the newborn.

4.30. A D E
A negative Coombs' test indicates there is no Rh isoimmunization. As the mother is already isoimmunized, anti-D gammaglobulin is of little use. In the absence of haemolysis, there is no cause for the baby to develop hyperbilirubinaemia. The rise in antibody titre during the pregnancy was non-specific and unrelated to the baby's Rh status. The only way to diagnose accurately the severity of Rh disease in the presence of rising antibody titre is by spectroscopic examination of amniotic fluid or fetal blood sampling.

4.31. E
A full-term infant has all the enzymes necessary for digestion of milk, iron therapy is not needed as the infant has adequate stores of iron derived from the mother. Subconjunctival haemorrhage usually occurs because of obstruction of venous return from the head and is not necessarily due to strangulation by cord around the neck. The aetiology of erythema toxicum is not known. The blood volume of a neonate is approximately 80–100 ml/kg.

4.32. B C E
In the presence of Rh isoimmunization of the mother anti-D gammaglobulin is of no use. Acidosis increases the penetration of CSF by bilirubin and thus increases the risk of kernicterus in the presence of hyperbilirubinaemia. As the antibodies are derived from the mother, blood of the mother's Rh group is suitable for exchange transfusion for it will not be haemolysed. The mother's blood will have positive indirect Coombs' test. Haemolysis continues after the neonatal period for a period of 6–12 weeks (half-life of gammaglobulin is 6 weeks).

4.33. Which of the following statements is/are true?
A Haemorrhagic disease of the newborn is a special risk of the first few days of neonatal life.
B The main complications of haemorrhagic disease of the newborn are intestinal and intracranial haemorrhage.
C Prophylactic vitamin K_1 should be given to all newborn babies.
D Vitamin K_1 administration is contraindicated in Rh incompatibility.
E Vitamin K_1 is contraindicated in the jaundiced newborn.

4.34. In the fetal circulation
A there is right-to-left shunting at atrial level.
B there is left-to-right shunting at ductal level.
C the pulmonary artery pressure is lower than the aortic pressure.
D oxygen saturation of the blood entering the fetal lung is lower than that of blood entering the aorta.
E persistence of blood flow through ductus arteriosus after delivery can be abolished by prostaglandin synthetase inhibitors.

4.35. Which of the following factors predispose(s) to the maintenance of a patent ductus arteriosus in the newborn?
A Prematurity.
B Respiratory distress syndrome of the newborn.
C Perinatal hypoxia.
D High fluid intake.
E Advanced maternal age.

4.36. Which of the following is/are correct regarding renal function in an infant born at 30 weeks' gestation?
A Glomerular filtration rate, corrected for surface area is less than in a normal adult.
B Nephron formation can be expected to continue for at least another 6 months.
C The ability to retain sodium is less than in a normal adult.
D Urinary concentrating ability is equal to that of a normal adult.
E A bladder catheter should be inserted if no urine has been passed by 24 hours of age.

4.33. A B C

Haemorrhagic disease is most common in the first few days of life because normally vitamin K_1 is derived from the gut organisms which are not present in the infant at birth. For this reason all newborn babies need prophylactic vitamin K_1. Bleeding may occur anywhere but is most serious when it occurs in the gastrointestinal tract (blood loss) or the central nervous system (brain injury). There is no contraindication to give vitamin K_1 in Rh incompatibility or a jaundiced newborn but synthetic vitamin K in large quantities would cause haemolysis and aggravate jaundice.

4.34. A D E

In the fetal circulation blood bypasses the lungs by getting across from the right atrium to the left atrium and from the pulmonary artery to the aorta due to high pulmonary artery pressure compared to the aortic pressures. Blood returning from the placenta is selectively directed towards the left atrium whereas that coming from the superior vena cava is directed towards the lung. Prostaglandin synthesis inhibitors such as indomethacin cause ductus arteriosus contraction and closure.

4.35. A B C D

The closure of the ductus arteriosus is caused by muscular contraction of the ductus due to high oxygen tension in the aorta. Conditions which affect these two factors will result in delayed closure. These include prematurity, respiratory distress syndrome and perinatal hypoxia. High fluid intake delays ductus closure but the mechanism is not clearly understood. Advanced maternal age does not affect ductal closure.

4.36. A C

Compared to an older child or adult the renal function is poor in the newborn. Glomerular filtration rate and the ability to concentrate sodium are diminished. Nephron maturation continues for months after birth but there is no new nephron formation. Babies may pass no urine in the first 24 hours of age (some of them may have passed at or before birth without it having been recorded) and therefore do not require catheterization.

4.37. Which of the following is/are true of neonatal urinary tract infection?
A   It is more common in twins.
B   It is commonly associated with fever and failure to thrive.
C   It may be complicated by neonatal meningitis.
D   It may be a factor contributing to neonatal jaundice.
E   It is more likely if the mother has a urinary tract infection.

4.38. Neonatal hypoglycaemia
A   does not occur in infants who have been fed early.
B   causes attacks of apnoea and cyanosis.
C   does not cause mental deficiency.
D   occurs more frequently in small-for-date infants than appropriate-for-date infants.
E   is defined as blood sugar level of less than 3.5 mmol/l.

4.39. The incidence of hypoglycaemia in the newborn is increased in
A   large-for-dates babies of diabetic mothers.
B   babies of mothers with pregnancy induced hypertension.
C   low birth weight babies for gestational age.
D   polycythaemia.
E   in infants with haemolytic disease in newborn due to Rh incompatibility.

4.40. In haemolytic Group B streptococcal infections in the first 5 days
A   the transmission of the organism is from the intrapartum exposure.
B   the treatment of choice is gentamicin.
C   virtually all infants develop meningitis.
D   at diagnosis the infant may appear deceptively well.
E   chest X-ray appearances are diagnostic.

4.37. C D E
The symptoms of neonatal urinary tract infection are non-specific. The commonest presentation is septicaemia or meningitis. Jaundice may be a prominent symptom. Infection is often acquired in utero especially if the mother has urinary tract infection. The incidence in twins is not increased.

4.38. B D
Early feeding will reduce the incidence of hypoglycaemia but will not prevent it in all infants. It can cause respiratory symptoms leading to cyanosis. Small-for-dates infants are more likely to develop hypoglycaemia because of their low glycogen reserves and their tendency to develop perinatal asphyxia. It is defined as a blood sugar level of less than 1.5 mmol/l in low-birth weight infants and less than 2.5 mmol/l in full-term infants.

4.39. A B C D E
Large-for-dates infants are born to diabetic mothers who are poorly controlled and have hyperinsulinaemia which results in hypoglycaemia. Small-for-dates babies are born to mothers with pregnancy-induced hypertension or intrauterine growth retardation. These babies have poor glycogen stores and are prone to hypoglycaemia. Polycythaemia results in hypoglycaemia due to increased metabolism of the red blood cells. Infants with haemolytic disease of newborn due to Rh incompatibility develop hypoglycaemia due to hyperinsulinism the exact mechanism of which is not known.

4.40. A D
Haemolytic Group B streptococcal infections are transmitted during parturition and can be prevented by administration of amoxycillin during labour. The organism is most sensitive to penicillin. Meningitis usually occurs in late onset disease. The disease is rapidly progressive though the infant may initially appear well. Chest X-ray appearances are non-specific and can be confused with hyaline membrane disease, aspiration pneumonias and transient tachypnoea of the newborn or may even be normal.

4.41. Which of the following statements on neonatal infections is/are true?

A   Hypothermia is a recognized sign of Gram-negative septicaemia.
B   Jaundice is a recognized sign.
C   Fresh human breast milk provides important protection against neonatal infections.
D   The incidence of neonatal infections could be reduced by having all newborn babies nursed in a single nursery.
E   Organisms normally regarded as commensals may cause serious disease in neonates.

4.42. Herpes simplex infection in the newborn

A   is usually due to type II virus.
B   causes jaundice before the third day of life.
C   usually requires speculum examination of the parturient mother for correct diagnosis.
D   is usually acquired during delivery.
E   responds promptly to intravenous cytosine arabinoside.

4.43. Congenital rubella infection has been associated with

A   cataract.
B   pleocytosis of the spinal fluid.
C   optic nerve hypoplasia.
D   diabetes mellitus.
E   deafness.

4.44. In congenital rubella

A   serum IgM is usually elevated at birth.
B   immunoglobulins IgG and IgM decrease from birth to 3 months.
C   the persistence of the infection is due to inability of the infant to produce antibodies against rubella.
D   ventricular septal defect is the commonest congenital heart lesion.
E   the infant is not infective after the age of 1 year.

4.41. A B C E
Neonatal infections rarely present with fever or localizing signs. Symptoms
are non-specific and include hypothermia and jaundice. Human breast milk
provides both cellular and humoral (IgA) protection against infections.
Neonatal infections are usually due to cross infection and would be reduced if
the nursery is small or preferably if the babies are nursed with their mothers.
Saprophytic organisms such as *Staphylococcus epidermidis*, *Pseudomonas
pyocyaneus* can cause serious infections in the newborn infant.

4.42. A B D
The type II virus accounts for about 75% of herpes simplex infections which
are acquired during delivery (following rupture of membranes). Diagnosis in
the mother is difficult and may not be obvious. Intravenous cytosine arabinoside has not been shown to be effective though treatment with acyclovir is
more encouraging. Jaundice is an early and prominent symptom.

4.43. A B D E
Congenital rubella infection causes cataract and glaucoma. Cataract is the
most characteristic ocular lesion of congenital rubella but may not be
recognized until after the neonatal period. CNS involvement is frequent and
may present with lethargy, irritability and bulging fontanelle. Spinal fluid
shows pleocytosis. The retina is involved but the optic nerve is spared.
Hearing loss may also manifest later in life which may be as late as school
age. Diabetes mellitus occurs many years later because of pancreatitis due to
the virus infection.

4.44. A
IgM does not cross the placenta and its presence at birth indicates a
congenital infection. In congenital infections (including rubella), there is
persistence of IgG because of continued infection. In congenital rubella the
infection persists as the body does not recognize the rubella virus as a foreign
substance and the viraemia persists for a number of years after birth. Patent
ductus arteriosus is the commonest congenital heart lesion.

4.45. **Which of the following infections may produce a clinical picture in the newborn resembling severe erythroblastosis fetalis?**

A   Cytomegalic inclusion disease.
B   *Pneumocystis carinii*.
C   Congenital syphilis.
D   Congenital listeriosis.
E   Gaucher's disease.

4.45. A C
Erythroblastosis fetalis is associated with conditions that cause intrauterine anaemia or infection. In this question A and C are therefore correct. *Pneumocystis carinii* and congenital listeriosis are acquired during delivery or are postnatal infections. Gaucher's disease does not cause any symptoms in the newborn.

5 Infection and immunology

5.1. Blood cultures are usually positive in cases of
A   supraglottic croup (epiglottitis).
B   campylobacter gastroenteritis.
C   whooping cough.
D   bronchiolitis.
E   bacterial meningitis.

5.2. Which of the following statements is/are true of *Streptococcus pyogenes* infections?
A   They account for less than 5% of upper respiratory infections in children under the age of 2 years.
B   The treatment of choice is ampicillin.
C   Rheumatic chorea is a recognized sequela.
D   It is a cause of erysipelas.
E   Penicillin prophylaxis is indicated for 2 years following acute nephritis.

5.3. Which of the following statements is/are true of meningococcal infections?
A   Penicillin is the drug of choice for chemoprophylaxis.
B   The meningococci can be cultured from the haemorrhagic skin lesions.
C   It is the commonest cause of meningitis in children under the age of 2 years.
D   Neurological sequelae are less likely following meningococcal meningitis than following other bacterial meningitis.
E   Blood cultures are rarely positive in the absence of skin lesions.

5.4. Which of the following statements is/are true of pertussis (whooping cough)?
A   Immunization is effective in preventing this disease in over 95% of immunized people.
B   For well premature infants the immunization should be carried out 2 months after birth.
C   Erythromycin has been shown to inhibit the growth of the aetiological agent in vitro.
D   Children under the age of 3 months are not at risk from the disease.
E   The incidence of permanent neurological complications from immunization is less than 0.1%.

5.1. A

Blood cultures are positive in supraglottic croup (the organism is *Haemophilus influenzae*) and in 70% of cases of bacterial meningitis. Bronchiolitis is a viral infection. *Bordetella pertussis* is cultured by a nasopharyngeal swab. *Campylobacter* is isolated by stool culture.

5.2. A C D

Most respiratory infections in children under the age of 2 years are viral in origin. The treatment of choice for streptococcal sore throat is penicillin. Rheumatic chorea may occur long after infection with streptococcus has resolved. Erysipelas which has a well-defined erythematous margin is due to streptococcal infection of dermis. Penicillin prophylaxis is not necessary following an attack of acute nephritis as second attacks are rare.

5.3. B D

Penicillin-resistant meningococci have been isolated and hence contacts of meningococcal disease should be given rifampicin till culture results are obtained. Other than epidemics, the commonenst cause of meningitis under the age of 2 years is *Haemophilus influenzae* and under the age of 1 month is *E. coli*. If diagnosed early, neurological sequelae after meningococcal meningitis are less common than other forms of meningitis. Blood cultures are positive in most cases even in the absence of skin lesions.

5.4. B C E

Newborn infants do not have transplacentally acquired immunity against pertussis and should be immunized as early as possible. Correct age is 2 months both for full-term and premature infants. Erythromycin has been shown to inhibit the growth of the organism in vitro. The incidence of permanent neurological complications is less than 1 in 150 000 cases.

5.5. In which of the following conditions is pertussis immunization contraindicated in a 2-month-old infant?
A   Baby exhibited neurological abnormalities in the neonatal period.
B   History of epilepsy in close relatives secondary to brain injury.
C   Family history of eczema.
D   Family history of cystic fibrosis.
E   Temperature of 38.5°C on routine examination at time of presentation for immunization.

5.6. Whooping cough
A   does not occur in the neonate if the mother has been previously immunized.
B   is more common is preschool than older children.
C   is contracted by droplet infection.
D   occurs around 21 days after exposure.
E   starts with a paroxysmal cough.

5.7. Which of the following statements is/are true of tuberculosis infection?
A   A 2-year-old Australian born child with positive tuberculin test who has no clinical disease requires antituberculous treatment.
B   BCG immunization has been proven to protect against miliary disease.
C   Atypical mycobacteria organisms usually cause pulmonary disease in childhood.
D   Chemotherapy is necessary only for three months.
E   Mortality rate from tuberculosis decreased significantly only when effective antituberculous drugs were introduced.

5.8. Which of the following statements about primary tuberculosis is/are correct?
A   The primary focus in the lung usually cavitates.
B   Symptoms from primary tuberculosis mostly arise from enlargement of the draining lymph nodes.
C   Some degree of blood-borne dissemination occurs with most cases of primary tuberculosis.
D   Sputum positive for AFB is required before making a diagnosis of primary tuberculosis.
E   Most cases of miliary tuberculosis and tuberculous meningitis occur within one year of initial infection with tuberculosis.

5.5. E

An acute illness (high fever) is a contraindication for immunization. None of the other conditions mentioned are absolute contraindication for pertussis immunization.

5.6. B C

Newborn infants do not have transplacentally acquired immunity against whooping cough. The incubation period of pertussis is 6–14 days and it is spread by droplet infection. The illness starts with a catarrhal stage which consists of rhinorrhoea, conjunctival injection, mild cough, wheezing and a low-grade fever. The incidence is highest in children under 5 years of age and 30% of cases occur in infants less than 6 months of age. Mortality is greatest in infants under 1 year of age.

5.7. A

Tuberculosis is rare in children born in Australia and a positive tuberculin test indicates that the child has been exposed to the tubercle bacillus. As there is a risk of generalized disease, treatment is indicated. BCG immunization results in primary infection which prevents generalized disease on reinfection. Atypical mycobacteria usually cause lymphadenitis. A 3-month course of chemotherapy for tuberculous infection is inadequate. Most patients require treatment for 6 months or longer. Mortality rates from tuberculosis decreased with improvement in housing and nutrition which decreased the spread of disease.

5.8. B C E

The primary lesion in the lungs usually heals leaving a small scar. The enlarged lymph nodes cause symptoms by pressure on bronchi. AFB are usually not isolated from the sputum in primary tuberculosis as there is no communication between the bronchi and the lung lesion. In primary tuberculosis the organisms are not localized to the site of infection and blood-borne dissemination occurs. Miliary tuberculosis and tuberculous meningitis can occur and usually do so within a year of initial infection.

5.9. The proper interpretation of a positive reaction to a tuberculin (Mantoux) test in a 9-year-old child is that the patient is
A   suffering from active tuberculosis.
B   immune to invasion by the tubercle bacillus.
C   susceptible to invasion by the tubercle bacillus.
D   in need of BDG vaccination.
E   sensitive to tuberculo-protein.

5.10. A child of 8 years has had a fever of 40°C (104°F) for 2 days. The tonsils are enlarged and inflamed and partly covered by a mucopurulent exudate. The cervical lymph nodes are enlarged and tender. Which of the following is/are true?
A   A negative Paul–Bunnell test would exclude glandular fever.
B   Hypertrophy of the lingual papillae and a confluent desquamating skin rash indicates haemolytic streptococcal infection.
C   If streptococci are grown from the throat swab, tetracycline is the treatment of choice in patients with penicillin allergy.
D   Palatal paralysis would indicate the need for immediate isolation.
E   Tonsillectomy should be advised following recovery.

5.11. Bacterial infection is the primary cause of
A   impetigo contagiosa.
B   seborrhoeic dermatitis.
C   psoriasis.
D   toxic epidermal necrolysis (scalded skin syndrome).
E   molluscum contagiosum.

5.12. Which of the following statements is/are true of *Herpes simplex* infection?
A   It can be transmitted sexually.
B   Primary infection is more severe than subsequent recurrence.
C   It is aggravated by exposure to the sun.
D   It often recurs in the same site.
E   It can be differentiated from other herpes viruses by electron microscopy.

5.9. E

A positive reaction to tuberculin indicates that the patient is sensitive to the tuberculo-protein which means the patient has been infected previously by the tubercle bacillus. It does not indicate active disease, immunity to tuberculosis or susceptibility to infection with the tubercle bacillus. BCG vaccination is contraindicated in these individuals.

5.10. B D

It is not unusual for the Paul–Bunnell test to be negative in glandular fever in children. Hypertrophy of the lingual papillae accompanied with a confluent desquamating rash suggests scarlet fever which is caused by beta-haemolytic streptococcal infection. The treatment of choice for streptococcal infections in patients with penicillin allergy is erythromycin. In the presence of palatal paralysis with the history in the stem one should suspect a diagnosis of diphtheria which requires isolation of the patient. There is no indication for tonsillectomy in this patient.

5.11. A D

Impetigo is caused by streptococcal and staphylococcal infections. Toxic epidermal necrolysis is a complication of staphylococcal infection. The aetiology of seborrhoeic dermatitis and psoriasis is not known. Molluscum contagiosum is caused by a virus.

5.12. A B C D

Herpes simplex infection can be transmitted sexually. In these cases the virus is identified most often to be Type 2. Approximately 85% of infections with *Herpes simplex* are asymptomatic. The symptoms are more severe with primary infection. The virus remains latent in neural tissue and can be reactivated by stress, exposure to the sun and tends to recur at the same site. It is a DNA virus and cannot be distinguished from other herpes viruses by electron microscopy.

5.13. Which of the following statements is/are true of *Mycoplasma pneumoniae* respiratory tract infections in children?

A   They are diagnosed by demonstrating cold agglutinins in the blood.
B   They are the most common cause of lower respiratory tract infections in children between 7–14 years.
C   The organism is easily grown from sputum cultures.
D   The infections are associated with middle ear disease.
E   They are treated with erythromycin.

5.14. A boy aged 7 months presents with a temperature of 39°C and irritability for 3 days. On the 4th day a generalized macular rash appears, the temperature subsides and then he is not irritable. Which of the following statements is/are true?

A   This presentation is typical of morbilli.
B   A positive diagnosis will be made by viral cultures of throat swabbing.
C   A possible diagnosis will be made by CSF examination.
D   This presentation is typical of roseola infantum.
E   This presentation is typical of drug allergy.

5.15. A woman in the 3rd month of pregnancy has been in contact the previous day with a known case of rubella. Which of the following statements is/are true?

A   If the haemagglutination-inhibition (HI) test is positive there is no risk to the fetus.
B   If the HI test is negative the mother should be immediately immunized with rubella vaccine.
C   If the HI test, initially negative, becomes positive a week later, natural immunity has developed and the fetus will be protected.
D   If the HI test remains negative throughout pregnancy and a healthy child is born no further action should be taken.
E   Demonstration of rubella-specific IgM one week later indicates recent infection.

5.16. Which of the following statements is/are true of infections with rubella virus?

A   Arthritis is a recognized complication.
B   The incubation period is 7–14 days.
C   Thrombocytopenia is a recognized complication.
D   Haemagglutination-inhibition antibodies are usually detected when rash appears.
E   Haemagglutination-inhibition antibodies persist longer than complement fixation antibodies.

5.13. B D E
Though cold agglutinins are increased in *Mycoplasma pneumoniae* infections, they are not diagnostic as they have been found in association with other viral respiratory infections. *Mycoplasma pneumoniae* may cause pneumonia in any age group but it most commonly affects adolescents and young adults. It may cause upper respiratory disease and has been isolated from patients with otitis media. The organism cannot be isolated from the sputum. Complement fixation is the best serological test for the diagnosis. The organism is sensitive to erythromycin and tetracycline.

5.14. D
Fever, irritability followed by a macular rash when the temperature subsides is diagnostic of roseola infantum. Throat swab cultures for viruses and CSF examination are not helpful in making a diagnosis. The white cell count shows leukopenia with relative lymphocytosis.

5.15. A E
A-positive haemagglutination-inhibition test indicates that the woman has had previous infection with rubella and therefore she is unlikely to get another attack of rubella and the fetus is at no risk of developing congenital rubella. Congenital rubella has been observed in infants following immunization with rubella vaccine during pregnancy. If the HI test becomes positive (being negative initially) it indicates that the mother has had a recent attack of rubella which places the fetus at risk of developing congenital rubella. If the HI test remains negative throughout pregnancy it means the mother is still at risk of developing rubella during subsequent pregnancies. She needs to be protected against this by active immunization following delivery. Following rubella infection, there is a rise in rubella-specific IgM which is diagnostic of the infection.

5.16. A C E
The incubation period of rubella is 14–21 days. Clinical manifestations include polyarthritis (usually of the hands) and thrombocytopenia. Haemagglutination-inhibition antibody titres appear in the convalescent stage and persist longer than complement fixation antibodies.

5.17. Which of the following is/are characteristic of measles?

A   Rhinitis.
B   Conjunctivitis.
C   Cough.
D   Enanthem.
E   Normal temperature when rash appears.

5.18. Which of the following is/are true of measles vaccine?

A   It is an inactivated virus.
B   It has an immune effect of at least 5 years.
C   It is unaffected in efficacy by any pre-existing measles antibody which has been passively or transplacentally acquired.
D   It gives better protection when injected at age 15 months than 9 months.
E   It is effective when given simultaneously with other immunizing agents.

5.19. Live measles vaccine is preferable to killed vaccine because it

A   does not require refrigeration.
B   does not cause any symptoms.
C   is less likely to cause atypical manifestations of infection.
D   can be given safely to immunodepressed patients.
E   does not require parenteral injection.

5.20. Live measles vaccine should NOT be given to children

A   with leukaemia.
B   on large doses of corticosteroids.
C   under the age of 3 months.
D   with eczema.
E   with history of convulsions.

5.17. A B C D
Rhinitis, conjunctivitis, cough and enanthem (Koplik spots) are manifestations of the prodromal phase of measles. The rash is often accompanied by high fever (40–40.5°C).

5.18. B D E
Measles vaccine consists of a live virus and its immune effect lasts at least 5 years. When given at 9 months it is likely to be less effective because of the neutralization of the vaccine by maternally-derived measles antibodies. The immunity will occur even when measles vaccine is given with other immunizing agents.

5.19. C
Both live and killed measles vaccine require refrigeration, may cause a measles-like illness and require a parenteral injection. Unlike killed vaccine, live vaccine should not be given to immunodepressed patients. Live vaccine is less likely to cause atypical manifestations of infection which include high fever, oedema of the extremities, pneumonitis and a haemorrhagic or urticarial rash over the extremities. Adverse reactions to measles vaccine include moderate fever which may occur during the month after vaccination. Usually fever, rash or both appear between the 5th and 12th days. Some children can occasionally develop febrile convulsions.

5.20. A B C
Live measles vaccine is contraindicated for patients who have immunosuppression which includes leukaemia and those receiving corticosteroids. It is not as effective if given to children under the age of 1 year and is inadvisable to be given to children under the age of 3 months. There is no contraindication for administering it to children with eczema or history of convulsions.

5.21. Comparing measles (morbilli) with German measles (rubella) it is a characteristic of the former that

A   the incubation period is longer.
B   the temperature period is longer.
C   pre-exanthem symptoms are of longer duration.
D   Koplik's spots appear.
E   suboccipital glands are more prominent.

5.22. Which of the following statements is/are true of chickenpox?

A   The patient is infective till all the scales have fallen.
B   Macules, papules, vesicles and scabs may be seen in different stages of development.
C   Pooled gammaglobulin can modify the course of disease in contacts.
D   Encephalitis is a recognized complication.
E   It is a recognized cause of calcification in the lungs.

5.23. Which of the following statements is/are true of threadworm infestation in children?

A   It is a common cause of anaemia.
B   It is transmitted directly from one child to another without an animal vector.
C   The threadworms migrate out through the anus to deposit their eggs on the perianal skin.
D   It is usually asymptomatic.
E   It is diagnosed by microscopy of stool specimen.

5.24. Which of the following is/are true concerning *Giardia lamblia* infestation in childhood?

A   Metronidazole is an appropriate therapeutic agent.
B   Stool microscopy is the most reliable diagnostic test.
C   It is a cause of intestinal disaccharide intolerance.
D   It does not occur in the first 4 weeks of life.
E   It is the cause of coeliac disease.

5.21. B C D
The incubation period of measles is 6–14 days, that of German measles is 14–21 days. The prodromal phase of rubella may go unnoticed whereas that of morbilli lasts 6–8 days and the fever persists and is maximum during the rash stage. Koplik spots are pathognomic of measles whereas suboccipital glands are more prominent in German measles.

5.22. B D E
In chickenpox the patient is infective 2 days before and 7 days after the onset of the rash and until all lesions are crusted. The lesions may be at different stages of maturity, i.e. macules, papules, vesicles and scabs may be seen simultaneously. Complications include encephalitis, secondary bacterial infection, thrombocytopenia, haemorrhagic lesions leading to purpura fulminans, myocarditis, pericarditis, myositis, hepatitis, glomerulonephritis, arthritis and Reye syndrome. Primary varicella pneumonia may be complicated by pleurisy with effusion and calcification in the lungs has been reported following chickenpox.

5.23. B C D
Threadworm infestation does not cause anaemia. Infection occurs by ingesting the eggs which are usually carried on fingernails, clothing, bedding or housedust or by autoinfection. The eggs are deposited by the worm on the perianal skin which results in perianal irritation and induces scratching though in the majority of cases there are no symptoms. Diagnosis is made by demonstrating the eggs on adhesive tape.

5.24. A C
Giardia lamblia infestation is best diagnosed by duodenal biopsy and examination of a wet preparation of intestinal mucosa. It causes lactose intolerance and responds to treatment with metronidazole. It can occur at any age and is not the cause of coeliac disease which is due to gluten enteropathy.

5.25. Toxoplasmosis is
A   a bacterial disease.
B   a cause of lymphadenitis.
C   usually lethal in man.
D   due to an organism that can cross the placental barrier.
E   resistant to treatment with sulphonamides.

5.26. Mumps
A   can be prevented by active immunization.
B   has a 2–3 week incubation period.
C   rarely affects the testes before puberty.
D   is rarely complicated by meningitis.
E   can cause nerve deafness.

5.27. In the infant of a woman with HIV infection which of the following is/are correct?
A   Transmission of HIV infection may take place during parturition.
B   Transmission of HIV infection during breast feeding has not been reported.
C   The risk of HIV infection in the infant is greater than 80%.
D   Failure to thrive may be the presenting symptom.
E   Diagnosis of HIV in the newborn infant cannot be made with routinely available tests.

5.28. Immunoglobulin G (IgG)
A   does not cross the placenta.
B   is the main immunoglobulin of external secretions.
C   is secreted by macrophages.
D   is the predominant serum immunoglobulin.
E   provides immunity against *Mycobacterium tuberculosis*.

5.25. B D

Toxoplasmosis is caused by *Toxoplasma gondii* which is a coccidian protozoa. It is an intracellular parasite which can multiply in all tissues of mammals and birds. Infection may be congenital when it may manifest like any other congenital infection or acquired which may be asymptomatic or present with malaise, fever, myalgia, maculopapular rash, localized or generalized lymphadenopathy, hepatomegaly, encephalitis, pneumonia, myocarditis and choroidoretinitis. Though the organism is sensitive to sulphonamides, a combination of pyrimethamine and sulphonamides is superior.

5.26. A B C E

Mumps immunization is carried out at the same age as measles and rubella immunizations, viz. 15 months. The incubation period of mumps is 2–3 weeks. Orchitis and epididymitis is rare in prepubescent boys but is common (14–35%) in adolescents and adults. Approximately 30–40% of affected testes atrophy. Though impairment of fertility is estimated to be about 10%, absolute infertility is rare. Meningoencephalitis is the most frequent complication in childhood (more than 65% of children show pleocytosis of cerebral spinal fluid). Unilateral nerve deafness may occur although the incidence is low (1 in 15 000). It is a leading cause of unilateral nerve deafness which may be transient or permanent.

5.27. A D E

Transmission of HIV infection from mother to infant can occur at birth through maternal blood and secretions. Infection has been reported to be acquired through breast milk. However, maternal AIDS is not a contraindication for breast feeding. Vertical transmission in utero occurs in 35–65% of cases. Common neonatal presentations include failure to thrive, lymphoid interstitial hyperplasia, opportunistic and bacterial infections, diarrhoea, hepatosplenomegaly and lymphadenopathy. Diagnosis in the newborn is difficult because HIV antibodies cross the placenta readily.

5.28. D

IgG crosses the placenta, and is the predominant serum immunoglobulin. It does not provide immunity against *Mycobacterium tuberculosis*. It is secreted by plasma cells which differentiate from B cells. The main immunoglobulin of external secretion is IgA.

5.29. In which of the following situations would you advise vaccination?
A   Triple antigen to a well premature infant at the age of 2 months.
B   Sabin vaccination in a child with recurrent Candida skin infections.
C   Hyperimmune gammaglobulin with hepatitis B vaccine to a newborn infant whose mother is HB surface antigen positive.
D   Smallpox vaccination for a child travelling to Indonesia.
E   Tetanus toxoid for a 2-year-old child with a penetrating builder's nail wound in the foot who is up to date with triple antigen vaccination.

5.30. Which of the following statements is/are true?
A   Pertussis vaccine should not be given to wheezing babies.
B   Sabin vaccine should not be given to immunosuppressed infants.
C   Atopy is not a contraindication to measles vaccination.
D   Rubella immunization of all girls in secondary schools will eliminate congenital rubella.
E   Premature infants should be given their first immunization at the chronological age of 2 months.

5.31. Which of the following statements regarding childhood immunization is/ are correct?
A   Polyarthritis is a recognized complication of rubella immunization.
B   Rubella immunization in childhood does not obviate the need for testing rubella immunity prior to conception.
C   A history of egg allergy is a contraindication to measles immunization.
D   A recent history of seizures is a contraindication to triple antigen.
E   Pertussis immunization reduces susceptibility to whooping cough by more than 95%.

5.32. Which of the following statements is/are true?
A   Triple antigen is given by subcutaneous injection.
B   A full course of immunization is adequate even if 3–4 months elapse between the first and second injections.
C   Sabin vaccine can be administered intramuscularly if the child vomits following oral administration.
D   Intraventricular haemorrhage in the newborn is not a contraindication for triple vaccine.
E   Severe adverse reactions to triple vaccine are thought to be due to diphtheria toxoid.

5.29. A C

Premature infants should be offered triple antigen at the chronological age of 2 months (i.e. the same as full-term infants). Hepatitis B antigen-positive mothers excrete the virus in all body secretions (milk, saliva) and are likely to infect their newborn infants which can be prevented by administration of hyperimmune gammaglobulin. Another tetanus toxoid injection is not required because immunity to tetanus following inoculation lasts 5–10 years. Recurrent Candida skin infection suggests disturbance of the T-cell function and is a contraindication for administration of live vaccine such as Sabin. Smallpox vaccination is not indicated for travel in any part of the world as the disease has been eliminated.

5.30. B C E

There is no contraindication for giving pertussis vaccine to wheezing babies or giving measles vaccination to atopic children. Live vaccines (which include Sabin) are contraindicated for immunosuppressed infants as they may develop clinical disease. Rubella immunization of all girls will not eliminate congenital rubella as the vaccination may not 'take' in all cases and in the presence of a susceptible population (boys) and unimmunized girls (those below the secondary school), rubella will be present in the community. Premature infants are immunized at the same chronological age as full-term infants, i.e. 2 months.

5.31. A B D

Clinical manifestations following rubella immunization include fever, lymphadenopathy, rash, arthritis and arthralgia. Rubella immunization offers protection in approximately 98% of cases. Though the immunity is lifelong there is evidence it may decrease gradually from which it follows that testing for immunity prior to conception is indicated. Though anaphylaxis following egg ingestion is a contraindication to measles immunization, egg allergy by itself is not a contraindication. As pertussis immunization has been implicated in the causation of neurological disease, its administration to a patient with a recent history of seizures may implicate it as the cause of an evolving neurological disease. Pertussis immunization is effective in 70–90% of cases.

5.32. B D

Triple antigen is given by deep intramuscular injection and is effective even if 3–4 months lapse between the first and second injections. Sabin vaccine can only be administered orally. Intraventricular haemorrhage in the newborn is not a contraindication for immunization with triple antigen (including pertussis vaccine). If severe reactions occur following the injection of triple antigen (in less than 1 in 150 000 cases) they are thought to be due to pertussis vaccine.

5.33. Which of the following statements is/are true?
A   Diphtheria toxoid is usually injected subcutaneously.
B   The diphtheria toxoid should be stored in the freezer compartment of the refrigerator.
C   CDT vaccine is contraindicated in children over 8 years.
D   Diphtheria antitoxin persists at protective levels for 10 years or more for those adequately immunized.
E   Sudden death can occur during convalescence from diphtheria.

5.34. Which of the following vaccines should NOT be administered during pregnancy and to patients with immunosuppression?
A   Whooping cough.
B   Oral polio (Sabin).
C   Rubella.
D   Measles.
E   BCG.

5.35. A 12-year-old girl was treated for membranous tonsillitis with penicillin and diphtheria antitoxin 17 days ago. Twelve days later she began to suffer intermittent fever, arthralgia and a transient blotchy rash with mild itching. The only clinical finding is generalized lymphadenopathy. She has microscopic haematuria and an elevated blood sedimentation rate. Further investigations will probably show
A   polymorphonuclear leucocytosis.
B   precipitating antibodies to bovine serum albumin.
C   a reduced total serum complement level.
D   elevated haemagglutination antibodies to equine gammaglobulin.
E   a positive LE cell preparation.

5.33. C D E
Diphtheria toxoid is injected intramuscularly. For children over 8 years, aluminium precipitate toxoid (APT) is recommended as combined diphtheria and tetanus toxoid (CDT) vaccine causes more adverse reactions. The vaccine is stored in the non-freezer compartment of the refrigerator. After immunization diphtheria and tetanus antitoxin persist at protective levels for 10 or more years. Sudden death during convalescence from diphtheria can occur due to myocarditis.

5.34. B C D E
Oral polio (Sabin), rubella, measles and BCG are live vaccines which may cross the placenta and infect the fetus. They are liable to cause frank disease in immunosuppressed patients. Hence they are contraindicated in these conditions. The vaccine of whooping cough is a dead organism and can be administered safely in pregnancy and to immunosuppressed patients.

5.35. A D
The history supports a diagnosis of serum sickness in which there is polymorphonuclear leucocytosis and elevated haemagglutination antibodies to equine gammaglobulin. There is no disturbance of the serum complement level or a positive LE cell preparation. There is no reason for the presence of precipitating antibodies to bovine serum albumin as the diphtheria antitoxin is usually prepared from equine serum by administering diphtheria toxoid to horses.

6 Gastrointestinal system

6.1. Swelling of the gums is significantly associated with which of the following conditions?
A   Scurvy.
B   Acute lymphoblastic leukaemia.
C   Hypothyroidism.
D   Phenytoin therapy.
E   Poor orodental hygiene.

6.2. Which of the following is/are true of gastro-oesophageal reflux?
A   It is associated with apnoeic spells.
B   It may present with respiratory distress.
C   It usually causes projectile vomiting.
D   Barium swallow and radiological screening will establish the diagnosis in all cases.
E   It may cause failure to thrive.

6.3. Which of the following statements is/are correct of gastro-oesophageal reflux in infancy?
A   Iron deficiency anaemia may be the presenting symptom.
B   Aspiration pneumonia is a complication.
C   The condition tends to improve spontaneously by 6–8 months of age.
D   Projectile vomiting is usually present.
E   It is often associated with cerebral palsy.

6.4. The symptoms and clinical findings in a newborn with oesophageal atresia WITHOUT FISTULA include
A   'mucusy' at birth.
B   cyanotic spells.
C   abdominal distension.
D   aspiration of gastric content if nursed supine.
E   meconium containing no hair.

6.1. A D E
Swelling of the gums occurs in scurvy due to bleeding (only if teeth have erupted), gum hypertrophy due to phenytoin therapy and infection due to poor orodental hygiene. It is not a feature of acute lymphoblastic leukaemia or hypothyroidism.

6.2. A B E
The apnoeic attacks are caused by reflex action because of acid in the oesophagus. Aspiration of the gastric contents will result in aspiration pneumonia and respiratory distress. Vomiting is usually effortless. Failure to thrive will result if the vomiting is persistent and in large amounts. As the reflux may be intermittent, barium swallow and radiological screening will not establish the diagnosis in all cases.

6.3. A B C E
In gastro-oesophageal reflux iron deficiency anaemia occurs due to reflux oesophagitis and bleeding. Aspiration pneumonia is due to the aspiration of stomach contents into the lungs. It tends to improve when the child adopts a sitting posture. Vomiting is usually effortless. The incidence is increased in patients with cerebral palsy.

6.4. A B E
The infant is 'mucusy' at birth because it is unable to swallow its saliva. Cyanotic spells occur due to the aspiration of the saliva into the trachea. Meconium does not contain hair as the fetus is unable to swallow amniotic fluid. Abdominal distension and aspiration of gastric contents cannot take place because there is no fistula between the oesophagus and trachea.

6.5. A 5-week-old infant presents with projectile vomiting of increasing severity for 10 days. He appears moderately dehydrated. The probable laboratory findings would be

A elevated blood pH.
B increased serum chloride.
C increased serum bicarbonate level.
D decreased urinary potassium level.
E low serum potassium level.

6.6. Which of the following is/are true of infantile hypertrophic pyloric stenosis?

A The narrowing of the lumen is principally due to hypertrophy of the longitudinal muscular layer.
B The onset is rare before the age of 1 week.
C The infant takes feeds hungrily.
D The vomitus usually contains bile.
E Small green frequent stools do not exclude the diagnosis.

6.7. In watery diarrhoea due to lactose intolerance

A Clinistix will detect the lactose in the stool.
B the stools will usually change blue litmus paper red.
C the diarrhoea will be fermentative (excess gas produced).
D the findings of 0.25% sugar in the stool strongly supports the diagnosis.
E for testing the stool is best collected off a nappy or bed sheet.

6.8. Chronic diarrhoea may be the presenting symptom of

A cystic fibrosis.
B lactose intolerance.
C blind loop syndrome.
D Meckel's diverticulum.
E coeliac disease.

6.5. A C E

Projectile vomiting of increasing severity in a 5-week-old infant is most likely to be due to pyloric stenosis which would result in loss of gastric fluid containing hydrochloric acid and potassium. This will result in raised blood pH, fall in serum chloride and increase in serum bicarbonate level. In order to maintain a normal pH, renal tubules will reabsorb hydrogen ions at the expense of excreting potassium ions in the urine which will result in an increased urinary potassium loss in spite of low serum potassium level.

6.6. B C E

In infantile hypertrophic pyloric stenosis the narrowing of the lumen is due to hypertrophy of the circular muscular layer. The onset is usually in the second to third week of life. As the stomach remains empty, the infant is hungry and feeds readily. The vomitus usually consists of gastric contents and contains no bile. The infant may have small green frequent stools which also occur in other conditions with starvation.

6.7. B C

Clinistix is specific for glucose and hence will not detect lactose. The stools are acid and will therefore turn litmus paper from blue to red. Lactose in the stool allows the gut organisms to ferment it. It is not uncommon for normal stools to contain up to 0.5% sugar. It is important to obtain the liquid part of the stool for testing and therefore it is better to collect it on a plastic sheet or obtain it by passing a soft rubber catheter into the rectum.

6.8. A B C E

Chronic diarrhoea occurs in cystic fibrosis because of lack of pancreatic enzyme, in lactose intolerance because of high osmolarity of lactose, in blind loop syndrome because of overgrowth of organisms and as a result of failure of absorption in coeliac disease (atrophic villi). Meckel's diverticulum causes no symptoms other than pain and bleeding.

6.9. Which of the following statements is/are correct of coeliac disease?
A   The clinical disease may be initiated by diet high in rye cereal.
B   The disease will usually affect either both or neither of two identical twins.
C   The condition has a self-limiting course and usually abates in late childhood.
D   The condition is diagnosed by assessing the clinical response to a gluten-free diet.
E   Typically during childhood the condition is associated with marked irritability.

6.10. Which of the following statements is/are correct in regard to coeliac disease?
A   The gluten-free diet should be continued throughout life.
B   There is an increased incidence in close relatives of affected children.
C   The malabsorption is due to pancreatic deficiency.
D   It is diagnosed on the basis of symptomatic response to a gluten-free diet.
E   Clinical onset is usually recognizable by 4 months of age.

6.11. In Crohn's disease of childhood
A   the terminal ileum is the most frequent site to be involved.
B   diarrhoea with blood and mucus is a characteristic early symptom.
C   growth retardation is a characteristic feature.
D   surgical resection of the affected gut is curative.
E   fever of unknown origin may be the presenting symptom.

6.12. Intussusception in childhood
A   may undergo spontaneous cure.
B   has, as the earliest sign, the passage of red-currant jelly stools.
C   has a peak incidence in the first 3 months of life.
D   requires operative reduction in the majority of cases.
E   may be started by a Meckel's diverticulum.

6.9. A E
Coeliac disease is caused by gluten (which is present in wheat and rye cereals). Studies have shown that though the disease is familial, there is discordance between monozygotic twins and only a 5% incidence in first-degree relatives. It is a life-long disease and is diagnosed by small bowel biopsy prior to introducing a gluten-free diet. One of the presenting symptoms in childhood is irritability.

6.10. A B
In coeliac disease gluten sensitivity is permanent and increases the risk of malignancy. Therefore the gluten-free diet should be continued throughout life. The condition is familial, the pancreatic secretion is normal. Diagnosis is based on demonstrating villous atrophy, regeneration of the villi following a gluten-free diet and recurrence of villous atrophy after reintroduction of gluten. Clinical onset does not occur for 3–4 months after the introduction of gluten in the diet.

6.11. A C E
As in adults, Crohn's disease in childhood affects the terminal ileum most frequently. Growth retardation and fever of unknown origin are the common presenting symptoms. Diarrhoea with blood and mucus are late symptoms. Surgical resection of the gut is not recommended unless there are complications such as perforation or intestinal obstruction.

6.12. A E
Intussesception may undergo spontaneous cure and may be started by a Meckel's diverticulum, though this is rare. Blood and mucus are late signs and may not appear at all. The peak incidence is at 6–8 months usually after weaning. Barium enema will confirm the diagnosis and can be used to reduce the intussusception in the majority of cases.

6.13. Intussusception in childhood is
A   most common in infants aged 6–9 months.
B   a self-limited condition.
C   more common in fat babies.
D   generally associated with a Meckel's diverticulum.
E   a recognized complication of Henoch–Schönlein purpura.

6.14. The treatment of a central umbilical hernia in a 4-month-old infant is
A   immediate surgical repair.
B   surgical repair at the age of 8 months.
C   application of a coin with adhesive tape.
D   reassurance of the mother.
E   none of the above.

6.15. Inguinal hernias
A   are more common than femoral hernias.
B   are more common in premature infants.
C   usually present with pain in the groin.
D   require an early elective operation.
E   require herniorrhaphy in children.

6.16. Which of the following statements related to infantile inguinal hernia is/ are correct?
A   Left-sided hernia is more common than right-sided hernia.
B   Inguinal hernia in a phenotypically female infant may contain testis.
C   The majority are direct.
D   An inguinal hernia associated with an undescended testis should be operated only when the neonate has reached the age suitable for orchidopexy.
E   The chance of bilateral hernias in a male infant is higher if he presents with a left rather than right hernia.

6.13. A C E

Typically intussusception occurs in well infants soon after weaning and progresses to gangrene of the bowel and shock. It is rarely associated with Meckel's diverticulum. In Henoch–Schönlein purpura the lead point is an intramural haematoma.

6.14. D

As the majority of umbilical hernias resolve spontaneously, the mother needs reassurance. If the problem persists beyond the age of 2 years the child may need an operation.

6.15. A B D

Femoral hernias are extremely rare in children. Incidence of inguinal hernias in premature infants is at least 3 times more than full-term infants. Inguinal hernias rarely cause pain. If pain is present in the groin it is much more likely to represent hip disease than hernia. Operation should be carried out as soon as possible as inguinal hernias in children tend to strangulate. Repair of inguinal hernia is carried out by high ligation of the sac. However, when a large internal inguinal ring exists, it is narrowed.

6.16. B E

In about 1% of phenotypically female infants the hernia may contain a testis. Such infants do not have a uterus and laparotomy reveals the absence of internal genital organs. Further investigations reveal that the infant has testicular feminization syndrome. Inguinal hernias are indirect, i.e. they follow the track of the descent of the testis. The hernias should be operated on as soon as possible after presentation as they are likely to strangulate. As the right testis descends after the left testis, it is more likely that the hernia will be present on the right side if it is present on the left which also accounts for a higher incidence of right-sided inguinal hernias.

6.17. Which of the following statements is/are true of diarrhoea and vomiting in infants?

A   Approximately 80% of cases in winter months are due to rotavirus.
B   It may be the presenting feature of urinary tract infection.
C   Hypernatraemic dehydration should be corrected within 12 hours of admission.
D   A normal potassium in serum indicates potassium chloride is not needed in the intravenous fluids.
E   Lactose intolerance is a common sequel in infants.

6.18. Which of the following methods of managment would you consider appropriate for gastroenteritis?

A   An electrolyte mixture containing 2% glucose for fluid replacement of a 2-year-old infant with 3–5% dehydration.
B   An electrolyte mixture containing 2% lactose for fluid replacement in an infant with mild rotavirus gastroenteritis.
C   A continuation of breast feeding with water between feeds for a 3-month-old baby with mild dehydration and watery diarrhoea containing greater than 2% reducing sugars.
D   A normal diet for a 3-year-old child with mild diarrhoea.
E   A low lactose (lactose hydrolysed milk based diet) for a 7-month-old breast-fed infant with 6% dehydration and reducing sugar positive fluid diarrhoea.

6.19. Which of the following statements regarding rotavirus diarrhoea in infants is/are correct?

A   Its incubation period is 48–72 hours.
B   Fever is a prominent feature.
C   Respiratory symptoms are present in about one-third to one-fourth of patients.
D   There is a greater water as compared to salt loss.
E   Breast feeding does not provide any protection.

6.20. Which of the following statements is/are true of gastroenteritis?

A   Lomotil will reduce the duration of the illness.
B   An infant under the age of 1 month should be admitted to hospital even though he may have mild symptoms.
C   Lactose intolerance if present is likely to be transient.
D   When due to *Salmonella typhimurium* it should be treated with amoxycillin or co-trimoxazole.
E   Anti-emetics are not recommended for children under the age of 5 years.

6.17. A B E
Rotavirus is the commonest organism causing gastroenteritis in winter months. Any parenteral infection (including urinary tract infection) in infants can present with diarrhoea. Hypernatraemic dehydration has to be corrected slowly over a period of 48 hours. In gastroenteritis there is a net loss of potassium and intravenous fluids should provide potassium. Following gastroenteritis there is destruction of the brush border of the small intestine which results in lactase deficiency and lactose intolerance for a period of 1–2 weeks.

6.18. A C D
Glucose in electrolyte solution helps in absorption of the fluid and electrolytes. Patients with gastroenteritis have lactose intolerance and therefore an electrolyte mixture containing lactose will aggravate the problem. Breast feeding with intermittent water between feeds will decrease the load of lactose. There is no need to change the diet in a 3-year-old with mild diarrhoea. Patients with 6% dehydration would need intravenous fluids.

6.19. A B C D
The incubation period of rotavirus diarrhoea is very short (48–72 hours). Fever and respiratory symptoms are prominent and the patient has profuse watery diarrhoea. Breast feeding provides little, if any, protection.

6.20. B C E
Medications have no place in treatment of gastroenteritis in infants. Lomotil will reduce the number of stools at the expense of pooling of fluid in the small intestine giving a false sense of security. Anti-emetics are usually not effective and also may cause side effects such as dystonia. Neonates require admission to hospital because of the risk of rapid deterioration and dehydration. The lactose intolerance is due to injury to the brush border of the small intestine which is replaced rapidly. Salmonella infections in infants are self-limiting. The administration of antibiotics results in prolongation of the carrier stage.

6.21. Which of the following statements is/are true of diarrhoea and vomiting?

A   Diarrhoea and vomiting in small infants do not necessarily indicate gastrointestinal infection.
B   Appendicitis can present as diarrhoea and vomiting.
C   Bacterial causes are readily distinguishable clinically from viral causes.
D   Breast feeding has been demonstrated to offer protection against infective diarrhoea and vomiting.
E   Lomotil is an accepted form of treatment in infants.

6.22. Development of abdominal distension in infants with gastroenteritis is suggestive of

A   hypocalcaemia.
B   hypokalaemia.
C   hyponatraemia.
D   intussusception.
E   endotoxaemia.

6.23. In which of the following conditions are fat droplets likely to be observed in the faeces?

A   Coeliac disease.
B   Sucrase-isomaltase deficiency.
C   Intestinal lymphangiectasia.
D   Pancreatic achylia (Schwachman's syndrome).
E   Biliary atresia.

6.24. A 2-month-old breast-fed infant is brought to see you because of persistent jaundice since birth. His stools are pale and his urine is highly coloured. Urine shows presence of bile but no urobilin. Which of the following is/are possible diagnosis/es?

A   Hypothyroidism.
B   Congenital viral infection.
C   Hereditary spherocytosis.
D   Congenital biliary atresia.
E   Breast milk jaundice.

6.21. A B D
Diarrhoea and vomiting in infants may be due to infection at other sites, due to ingestion of 'poisons', and may be a presenting symptom of appendicitis. It is not possible clinically to distinguish between bacterial and viral causes of gastroenteritis. The protection against infective diarrhoea due to breast feeding is thought to be due to the presence of IgA in the milk. Lomotil has no place in the treatment of gastroenteritis in infants.

6.22. B D E
Hypocalcaemia and hyponatraemia do not cause disturbance of intestinal motility. In hypokalaemia and endotoxaemia there is ileus which results in abdominal distension. The abdominal distention in intussusception (which is a complication of gastroenteritis) is caused by intestinal obstruction.

6.23. D E
In pancreatic achylia there is deficiency of pancreatic enzymes including lipase which results in failure of digestion of fat. In biliary atresia fat droplets appear in the stool because the process of absorbing whole fats by emulsification is inhibited. In coeliac disease and intestinal lymphangiectasia though there is steatorrhoea, there are no fat droplets in stools.

6.24. B D
This patient has obstructive jaundice which occurs in congenital viral infections and congenital biliary atresia. The jaundice of hypothyroidism, hereditary spherocytosis and breast milk is not obstructive.

110

6.25. Which of the following statements regarding hepatitis B is/are true?
A   It may be acquired by the faecal-oral route.
B   Hepatitis B surface antigen can usually be identified in the first week of the illness.
C   Persistence of the antigenaemia for more than 3 months after the acute attack may be associated with chronic liver disease.
D   The incubation period is 4 weeks.
E   Newborn infants whose mothers have hepatitis B surface antibodies require hyperimmune gammaglobulin for prophylaxis.

6.26. Which of the following statements is/are true?
A   Six to eight watery, yellow stools daily with curds are within the normal range for breast-fed infants.
B   Breast-fed infants who pass no stools for 3 days require a laxative.
C   The presence of 0.5% lactose in stools of a breast-fed baby usually requires no treatment.
D   Breast-fed babies do not develop cow's milk allergy.
E   The presence of greenish, grey stools in a bottle-fed (commercial formula) baby requires further laboratory investigations.

6.27. Acute anal fissure is
A   associated with pain on defaecation.
B   a cause of bright blood streaks on surface of motion.
C   a recognized feature of Crohn's disease.
D   best treated by surgical excision.
E   associated with constipation.

6.28. Which of the following statements is/are true of Hirschsprung's disease?
A   The rectum is usually empty.
B   The symptoms may be mild while the child is fully breast-fed.
C   The dilated portion of the gut shows absence of parasympathetic ganglia.
D   The incidence is higher in infants who have meconium plugs at birth.
E   It is rarely present in premature infants.

6.25. A B C
Though commonly acquired by injection of contaminated body fluids, hepatitis B can be acquired by faecal oral route. The hepatitis B surface antigen can be identified in serum soon after the onset of illness. Its persistence leads to chronic liver disease. The disease has an incubation period of more than 6 weeks. The presence of surface antibodies indicates that the person has immunity to hepatitis B. Such persons are not carriers (or infective) and their contacts do not require passive immunization.

6.26. A C
It is normal for breast-fed infants to pass 6–8 stools a day or 1 stool in a week. Their stools contain up to 0.5% lactose. Breast-fed infants can develop cow's milk allergy because of the passage of cow's milk protein through breast milk. Greenish, grey stools in bottle-fed babies are due to the iron in the formula.

6.27. A B C E
Acute anal fissure is painful and causes spasm of the anal sphincter which results in pain on defaecation. The problem usually starts with constipation. The stools are blood streaked as bleeding occurs during defaecation. Anal fissure is a common complication of Crohn's disease. Surgical excision is rarely required.

6.28. A B D E
In Hirschsprung's disease, because of lack of peristalsis, the aganglionic segment is narrow and empty and the proximal portion of the gut is dilated. It may present as a meconium plug at birth. It has been shown to be rare in premature infants. Low residue in breast milk may account for the delay in onset of symptoms.

7 Respiratory system

7.1. Arterial hypoxaemia in acute asthma
A may be unchanged despite improvement in FEV_1 in the acute phase.
B is usually associated with hypercapnia.
C may occur in the absence of rhonchi on auscultation.
D may worsen after intravenous aminophylline.
E need not be associated with cyanosis.

7.2. Pulmonary oedema occurs in which of the following?
A Smoke inhalation in a fire.
B Transfusion reaction.
C Sea water drowning.
D Heart failure complicating isolated pulmonary stenosis.
E Pneumonia.

7.3. Pulmonary function tests in a child with moderately severe asthma are likely to show
A increased vital capacity.
B increased functional residual capacity.
C normal timed vital capacity (FEV_1).
D decreased vital capacity.
E increased tidal volume.

7.4. Accepted indications for the removal of adenoids in childhood are
A mouth breathing.
B serious postnasal obstruction.
C nasal escape of air in speech.
D snoring.
E recurrent otitis media.

7.1. C D E
Improvement in FEV_1 in acute asthma results in improvement of arterial oxygen tension. Hypoxia usually precedes hypercapnia. Rhonchi will not be heard in asthma if air entry is poor. It has been demonstrated that arterial oxygen tension falls following intravenous aminophylline due to disturbance of pulmonary perfusion. Cyanosis is a poor sign for arterial hypoxaemia as it does not occur till the oxygen saturation has dropped below 75%.

7.2. A B C
Pulmonary oedema in smoke inhalation occurs due to damage of the alveoli, in transfusion reactions due to heart failure and sea water drowning due to osmosis (sea water is hypertonic, equivalent to 3% saline). In pneumonia there is an exudate. In heart failure due to pulmonary stenosis there is no pulmonary oedema.

7.3. B D
In severe asthma vital capacity, FEV_1 and tidal volume are decreased whereas residual lung volume is increased.

7.4. B
Serious postnasal obstruction due to enlargement of the adenoids is an absolute indication for adenoidectomy. This can be demonstrated by a lateral X-ray of the postnasal space. Not often the mouth-breathing is due to causes other than enlarged adenoids, e.g. mucosal thickening due to allergy. Nasal escape of air is an absolute contraindication to the removal of adenoid tissue. Snoring, unless related to enlargement of adenoids, is not an indication for adenoidectomy. There is much debate as to whether adenoids should be removed from children who suffer from recurrent middle ear disease; the anatomical linkage of the postnasal space with the middle ear by the Eustachian tube is an enticing argument, but proof by statistical means is lacking.

7.5. The accepted indications for the removal of tonsils in childhood are

A   peritonsillar abscess.
B   frequent serious upper respiratory tract infections requiring frequent absences from school.
C   eight or more attacks of tonsillitis per year despite chemoprophylaxis.
D   sleep apnoea.
E   recurrent middle ear infections.

7.6. Tonsillitis due to streptococcal infection can be differentiated from tonsillitis of other aetiology by

A   the presence of exudate on the tonsils.
B   the magnitude of cervical lymph node enlargement.
C   white cell count of greater than 15 000 per cmm.
D   the size of the tonsils.
E   none of the above.

7.7. Which of the following statements is/are likely to be true of acute otitis media?

A   May have fever as the only presenting feature.
B   Light reflex is altered.
C   Decongestive agents have been demonstrated to be efficacious.
D   Drug of choice for treatment is penicillin.
E   Most infections are bacterial in origin.

7.8. Which of the following statements is/are true about glue ear?

A   More than 30% of all children at some time have seromucus fluid in a middle ear (glue ear).
B   The prevalence of glue ear drops sharply by mid-primary school age.
C   Ventilating tubes are indicated for children with glue ear having low frequency hearing loss of 30 dB with normal hearing for middle and high frequency.
D   Intermittent hearing loss with head colds in a child with a mild glue ear problem is an indication for inserting ventilating tubes.
E   The amount of scarring of the eardrum depends more on the severity of the middle ear problems than on the frequency of the insertion of ventilating tubes.

7.5. A B D

Frequent attacks of real tonsillitis despite appropriate antibacterial prophylaxis is accepted as an indication for tonsillectomy by even the most conservative paediatricians; however, the emphasis is on *real* tonsillitis and not just the tonsils inflamed as part of an upper respiratory tract infection due to viral causes which are not an indication no matter how severe they may be. Peritonsillar abscess previously was regarded as an absolute indication but effective use of appropriate antibiotic therapy with surgical drainage where indicated, has produced cure so that in many, perhaps most cases, tonsillectomy is no longer necessary. Sleep apnoea is an absolute indication. There is no association between the tonsils and middle ear infection.

7.6. E

The only way to distinguish between viral and bacterial tonsillitis is by culture of a throat swab.

7.7. A B

In acute otitis media fever and irritability are the main symptoms though irritability is not always present. The landmarks of the ear drum are not clear and the light reflex is altered. Decongestive agents are of little use. Most infections are viral in origin. The drug of choice is amoxycillin or trimethoprim with sulphamethoxazole as the infecting organisms are *Haemophilus influenzae*, *Streptococcus pyogenes* or *Streptococcus pneumoniae*.

7.8. A B E

Glue ear of minor severity is often symptomless and has been observed in more than 30% of children at some time. Its prevalence (and the incidence of acute otitis media) drops sharply by mid-primary school age. Low frequency hearing loss of 30 dB is not a significant hearing handicap for children, does not cause irreversible damage and requires no treatment. Provided that there is little handicap at other times, obvious deafness with head colds (which lasts for a few days) is not an indication for ventilating tubes. Tympanic membrane scarring is largely dependent on severity of middle ear disease.

7.9. Which of the following is/are true regarding acute epiglottitis due to *Haemophilus influenzae*?

A   It occurs only in children.
B   *Haemophilus influenzae* type B is rarely cultured from the blood.
C   Drooling is due to palatal paralysis.
D   Examination of the throat in your surgery is the diagnostic procedure.
E   Family contacts under the age of 4 years should be treated with rifampicin.

7.10. Acute epiglottitis is associated with

A   gradual onset of cough, fever and stridor over several days.
B   infection with parainfluenza virus.
C   *Haemophilus influenzae* type B septicaemia.
D   drooling and difficulty in swallowing.
E   high probability of recurrence.

7.11. In laryngomalacia there is characteristically

A   micrognathia.
B   inspiratory stridor.
C   difficulty in feeding.
D   tendency to improvement with age.
E   predisposition to croup.

7.12. Which of the following is/are true of acute laryngotracheobronchitis (croup)?

A   Barking cough and hoarse voice are early symptoms.
B   Boys are more likely to be admitted to hospitals than girls.
C   The symptoms frequently respond to salbutamol.
D   The use of nebulized adrenaline is contraindicated.
E   Parainfluenza viruses are the predominant aetiological agents.

7.9. E

Though most common in the age group 5–10 years, acute epiglottitis can occur at any age. Blood culture usually reveals *Haemophilus influenzae*. The patient is unable to swallow because of the swelling of the epiglottis. As some patients stop breathing during examination of the throat because of impaction of epiglottic folds between the 'true' cords it should not be undertaken unless facilities for intubation are available. Family contacts under the age of 4 years need prophylaxis with rifampicin because they may contract the disease.

7.10. C D

The onset of acute epiglottitis is sudden. *Haemophilus influenzae* is the causative agent and can be cultured from the blood. The patient has difficulty in swallowing which is due to the swollen epiglottis which results in drooling. Recurrence risk is low.

7.11. B C D E

There is no association between laryngomalacia and micrognathia. The inspiratory stridor is due to partial closure of the larynx during inspiration which results in difficulty with feeding. The symptoms improve with age because the larynx gets bigger in all directions. Infections result in decrease in circumference of the larynx (due to oedema) which manifests as croup.

7.12. A B E

The characteristic features of croup are barking cough and hoarse voice which are worse at night than during the day. The disease appears to be more severe in boys. Parainfluenza viruses are the predominant aetiological agents. It does not respond to treatment with salbutamol by nebulizer though it may show response to adrenaline by nebulizer.

7.13. Which of the following clinical features is/are characteristic of severe bronchiolitis in infants?
A   Restlessness.
B   Insidious onset.
C   Cyanosis.
D   Loss of liver dullness to percussion.
E   Respiratory acidosis.

7.14. In acute bronchiolitis in a 6-month-old infant
A   the neutrophil count is a good guide to aetiology.
B   oxygen should be used cautiously because of danger of producing hypercapnia.
C   *Haemophilus influenzae* is the commonest pathogen.
D   antibiotic treatment has been demonstrated to be effective.
E   respiratory rate and excursion are useful guides to severity of illness.

7.15. Over the period of a day, a 4-month-old infant develops tachypnoea, chest recession, widespread crepitations and expiratory rhonchi. Chest X-ray suggests hyperinflation of the lungs. Which of the following statements is/are correct?
A   Viral studies would show presence of a rhinovirus in 25% of cases.
B   The infant has more than a 20% chance of becoming asthmatic later in life.
C   Significant improvement is likely to be obtained by treatment with salbutol by inhalation.
D   Corticosteroid treatment improves the mortality rate in such cases.
E   The parents may be reassured that the critical period of his illness will not have a duration of more than 48 hours.

7.16. Which of the following statements is/are true of asthma in children?
A   It may present with nocturnal cough without wheeze.
B   It is usually ameliorated by desensitizing injections.
C   If it is exercise induced it is usually worse after swimming than running.
D   Exercise-induced asthma can be prevented by salbutamol inhalation prior to exercise.
E   Children are less likely to grow out of it if there is a family history of atopy.

7.13. A B C D E

Bronchiolitis has an insiduous onset and results in hyperexpansion of the lungs which causes loss of liver dullness to percussion. It is accompanied by hypoxia which results in restlessness and cyanosis, and hypercapnia which results in respiratory acidosis.

7.14. E

In acute bronchiolitis the neutrophil count is variable. There is no danger in administering oxygen as the condition is of acute onset. Respiratory syncytial virus is the commonest causative organism and therefore antibiotics have no effect on the course of the disease. The respiratory rate and excursion indicate the severity of the disease.

7.15. B

The history suggests a diagnosis of bronchiolitis. The rhinoviruses usually cause infections of the nose and rarely cause bronchiolitis. Epidemiological studies have shown that about a third of patients with bronchiolitis develop asthma later in life. Bronchodilators and corticosteroids do not affect the course of the disease. Though in most cases the disease is most severe for the first 48 hours, death can occur after this period.

7.16. A D E

A reactive airway (asthma) commonly presents with cough at night. Wheezing may not be present. Many agents have been implicated in the causation of asthma and therefore desensitization is almost impossible. The main trigger in exercise-induced asthma is dry air which is less likely to be encountered while swimming. Prior inhalation of salbutamol will prevent exercise-induced asthma by maintaining bronchodilatation. The prognosis for childhood asthma is good though the asthma is more likely to persist and be severe with a family history of atopy.

7.17. In the treatment of acute asthma
A i.v. aminophylline may exacerbate hypoxia.
B the effect of i.v. hydrocortisone is maximal in one hour.
C ipratropium bromide is contraindicated.
D sodium cromoglycate (Intal) is only of use as a prophylactic agent, and cannot control the acute attack.
E antibiotics should be used prophylactically.

7.18. A foreign body in the respiratory passage can cause
A atelectasis.
B unilateral pulmonary hyperinflation.
C mediastinal displacement.
D wheezing.
E recurrent chest infection.

7.19. Which of the following statements is/are true of aspiration of a foreign body?
A The symptoms associated with aspiration vary with the area of entrapment.
B A large number of aspirated foreign bodies are foods.
C The highest risk age group is in children aged 4–6 years.
D Foreign body aspiration should be considered as a possible cause of cough/wheeze in a 2-year-old child even when no history of aspiration is obtained.
E Foreign bodies are usually radio-opaque.

7.20. In acute bronchopneumonia in a 6-month-old infant
A the neutrophil count is a good guide to aetiology.
B oxygen should be used cautiously because of the danger of producing hypercapnoea.
C *Streptococcus pyogenes* is the commonest pathogen.
D tetracycline is the most satisfactory antibiotic for initial therapy.
E respiratory rate and excursion is a useful guide to severity of illness.

7.17. A D
In the treatment of acute asthma i.v. aminophylline exacerbates hypoxia by decreasing pulmonary perfusion, i.v. hydrocortisone is not effective till 4–6 hours after injection, ipratropium bromide acts synergistically with other bronchodilators and prophylactic antibiotics are not indicated as infection if present is usually viral. Sodium cromoglycate is a prophylactic agent and may exacerbate an acute attack.

7.18. A B C D E
The presenting symptoms of foreign body in the respiratory passage depends on whether it causes complete or incomplete obstruction and its location in the respiratory tree. Complete blockage results in atelectasis. Incomplete blockage results in hyperinflation, wheezing and mediastinal displacement to the opposite side. Recurrent chest infection usually occurs with complete blockage.

7.19. A B D
Symptoms of foreign body aspiration include acute apnoea if the foreign body is lodged in the larynx or trachea, severe respiratory distress if the foreign body is lodged in a major bronchus, wheezing when the obstruction is partial, signs of consolidation when there is superadded infection. Most foreign respiratory bodies are food (and therefore are not radio-opaque) and occur in children below the age of 4 years.

7.20. E
Acute bronchopneumonia is usually due to a bacterial infection. The neutrophil count would suggest such a diagnosis but would not identify the organisms. The commonest pathogen is *Haemophilus influenzae*. There is no contraindication for administering oxygen as the condition is of acute onset and there is no danger of respiratory arrest. Tetracycline is not recommended for infants as it stains the teeth. The more severe the disease the more likely the respiratory rate and excursion will be increased and vice-versa.

7.21. The ultimate outcome in healthy children who survive staphylococcal pneumonia is usually
A   recurrent spontaneous pneumothoraces.
B   chronic respiratory insufficiency.
C   chronic lung abscesses and empyema.
D   persistent pneumatoceles.
E   complete resolution.

7.22. A previously well 5-year-old boy presents with a two-week history of cough, malaise and low grade fever. He has been treated by his local medical officer with amoxycillin with no improvement. Auscultation of his chest reveals widespread crepitations and a chest X-ray shows an interstitial generalized infiltrate. Which of the following statements is/are true?
A   The picture is consistent with viral pneumonitis.
B   The most likely cause is infection with amoxycillin-resistant *Haemophilus influenzae*.
C   Asthma is the likely diagnosis.
D   Positive cold agglutinins will be diagnostic of mycoplasma pneumonitis.
E   The picture is consistent with staphylococcal pneumonia.

7.23. Recurrent respiratory tract infections have significant association with
A   ventricular septal defect.
B   tetralogy of Fallot.
C   gastro-oesophageal reflux.
D   parental smoking.
E   attendance at playschool.

7.24. Which of the following statements is/are true of fibrocystic disease of the pancreas?
A   Intestinal disaccharidase levels are low.
B   Prognosis is unchanged even with optimal management.
C   There is an incidence of 1 in 4 of this condition in the offspring of unaffected siblings.
D   There is an increased incidence of neonatal bowel obstruction.
E   Neonatal screening for immunoreactive trypsin will establish early diagnosis in 98% of cases.

7.21. E
In the acute phase, staphylococcal pneumonia could result in recurrent spontaneous pneumothoraces and empyema, lung abscesses and persistent pneumatoceles. Long-term follow-up will show complete resolution. Chronic respiratory insufficiency is not a feature of staphylococcal pneumonia.

7.22. A
Insiduous onset with persistent symptoms, and widespread changes in the lung with the mildness of the illness suggest a diagnosis of viral pneumonitis rather than a bacterial infection. Clinical history and physical findings are inconsistent with the diagnosis of asthma. While a rise in cold agglutinins titre is suggestive of a diagnosis of mycoplasma pneumonitis it is not diagnostic.

7.23. A C D E
Recurrent respiratory tract infections occur in ventricular septal defect due to pulmonary congestion, in gastro-oesophageal reflux because of aspiration, attendance at playschool because of exposure to other children's infection. Epidemiological studies have shown that parental smoking increases the incidence of recurrent respiratory tract infections. In tetralogy of Fallot there is pulmonary ischaemia and there is no increased incidence of recurrent respiratory tract infection.

7.24. D
In cystic fibrosis there are no changes in intestinal disaccharidase levels. Over the last 20 years the life expectancy of cystic fibrosis patients has increased from 10 to more than 20 years. The incidence in the offspring of unaffected siblings is approximately 1 in 300 ($\frac{1}{3} \times \frac{1}{4} \times \frac{1}{25}$). Neonatal bowel obstruction is usually due to meconium ileus or may be due to ileal atresia with or without meconium peritonitis. Neonatal screening with immunoreactive trypsin gives both false positive and false negative results.

7.25. Cystic fibrosis is recognized as being associated with

A   meconium ileus.
B   malabsorption.
C   hypertension.
D   rectal prolapse.
E   growth retardation.

7.26. Which of the following statements is/are true of cystic fibrosis?

A   The absence of fat in stools excludes the diagnosis.
B   Heterozygotes can be identified by the sweat test.
C   Males are usually sterile.
D   Intestinal obstruction may be a presenting symptom in the newborn.
E   Life expectancy is less than 20 years.

7.27. In cystic fibrosis

A   the heterozygote frequency is closer to 1 in 25 than 1 in 100.
B   failure to thrive is due to pancreatic insufficiency alone.
C   the high sweat sodium content is of no clinical significance other than for diagnosis.
D   rectal prolapse is a recognized mode of presentation.
E   physiotherapy is an essential component of management.

7.25. A B D E

In cystic fibrosis, meconium ileus and malabsorption are due to absence of pancreatic enzymes; growth retardation and rectal prolapse are due to malabsorption. Hypertension is not a feature of cystic fibrosis.

7.26. C D

In cystic fibrosis heterozygotes cannot be identified by the sweat test; males are sterile because of the abnormalities of the vas deferens. It may present with intestinal obstruction due to meconium ileus in the newborn. Presently the life expectancy is more than 20 years. Though fat is usually present in the stools, its absence does not exclude the diagnosis.

7.27. A D E

The incidence of cystic fibrosis is 1 in 2500. The heterozygote frequency is 1 in 25. Failure to thrive is due to pancreatic insufficiency and recurrent respiratory tract infections which require physiotherapy. The high sweat sodium content can lead to hyponatraemia. Rectal prolapse is a recognized mode of presentation in infancy.

8 Cardiovascular system

8.1. The innocent (physiological) systolic murmur in an 8-year-old child
A   usually changes intensity with posture.
B   is inaudible posteriorly.
C   is maximal in the 4th/5th left interspace.
D   may be associated with a third heart sound.
E   can be musical or high pitched in character.

8.2. The interval between aortic and pulmonary valve closure sounds is increased on inspiration in the normal patient because of
A   descent of the diaphragm.
B   prolongation of left ventricular systole.
C   sinus arrhythmia.
D   prolongation of right ventricular systole.
E   a rise in pulmonary artery pressure.

8.3. A previously well 3-month-old infant presents with reluctance to feed and breathlessness. A pulse rate of 250/min is obtained. Which of the following statements is/are correct?
A   The most likely diagnosis is supraventricular tachycardia.
B   The infant does not require any treatment immediately.
C   If physical measures fail to slow the heart rate, digitalis should be administered.
D   A normal QRS complex precludes the diagnosis of Wolff–Parkinson–White syndrome.
E   The long-term prognosis is good.

8.4. In which of the following conditions is pulsus paradoxus likely to be present?
A   Pericardial effusion.
B   Rheumatic pericarditis.
C   Pneumothorax.
D   Asthma.
E   Cardiac failure.

8.1. A B D E
The innocent systolic murmur is heard in more than 30% of children. It is ejection, musical (frequently sounding like the vibration of a tuning fork), brief in duration, may be attenuated in the sitting position and is intensified by fever, excitement or exercise. It is best heard along the left lower and midsternal border or the pulmonary area. It does not radiate to the back, base or apex of the heart.

8.2. D
During inspiration right ventricular ejection time increases due to increased filling of the heart which increases the interval between the aortic and pulmonary valve closure sounds.

8.3. A C E
A pulse rate of more than 200/min with reluctance to feed and breathlessness support a diagnosis of supraventricular tachycardia with cardiac failure which needs active treatment and will respond to treatment with digitalis. If treated adequately the long-term prognosis is good. Between the attacks some infants demonstrate ECG changes of Wolff–Parkinson–White syndrome.

8.4. A C D
In pericardial effusion there is pulsus paradoxus because of decreased filling of the left side of the heart during inspiration. In pneumothorax and asthma the pulsus paradoxus is due to increased intrathoracic pressure. In rheumatic pericarditis and cardiac failure there is no change in filling of the heart between inspiration and expiration.

8.5. An otherwise well 3-year-old boy undergoing routine physical examination is repeatedly found to have a blood pressure of 120/90 mmHg when using a cuff covering most of the upper arm. Which of the following is/are appropriate?

A   Take the blood pressure again using a smaller cuff.
B   Measure lower limb blood pressures.
C   Review in 1 year.
D   Measure plasma cholesterol and triglyceride levels.
E   Admit child to hospital urgently.

8.6. Causes of systolic hypertension in children include

A   coarctation of the aorta.
B   patent ductus arteriosus.
C   acute urinary tract infection.
D   acute glomerulonephritis.
E   neuroblastoma.

8.7. In blood pressure recording

A   the width of the cuff should be two-thirds (or more) of the length of the upper arm.
B   the average pressure in late infancy is approximately 80/55 mmHg by auscultation.
C   the flush pressure approximates to the systolic value.
D   measurement over the lower limbs is more reliable than over the upper limbs.
E   the patient's posture (sitting or supine) has no effect on the measurement.

8.8 Right ventricular hypertrophy is

A   a characteristic feature of transposition of great vessels.
B   a characteristic feature of tetralogy of Fallot.
C   a characteristic feature of tricuspid atresia.
D   diagnosed when the T wave is upright in V1 after 72 hours of age.
E   diagnosed when R in V1 exceeds 20 mm.

8.5. B E
The patient has a very high blood pressure which may lead to hypertensive encephalopathy or renal failure. He requires urgent admission and further investigations. The high blood pressure may be due to coarctation and hence measurement of blood pressure in the lower limbs is useful in establishing the diagnosis. A smaller cuff will give an erroneously high blood pressure. There is no indication for measuring serum cholesterol and triglyceride levels.

8.6. A B D E
Coarctation of the aorta and acute glomerulonephritis cause high blood pressure due to disturbance of blood supply to the kidneys. In patent ductus arteriosus the systolic blood pressure is raised because of increased cardiac output. In neuroblastoma the raised blood pressure is due to catecholamines. Acute urinary tract infection does not cause disturbance in blood pressure.

8.7. A B C
For accurate measurement of blood pressure the width of the cuff should be two-thirds to three-quarters of the length of the upper arm. Measurement of blood pressure by the flush method gives approximately the systolic value as blood begins to flow as soon as the cuff's pressure is below the systolic level. The blood pressure at term is 70/50 mmHg. It gradually increases with advancing age reaching a value of 120/75 by the age of 16 years. Blood pressure is affected by posture.

8.8 A B D E
Right ventricular hypertrophy occurs in transposition of great vessels and tetralogy of Fallot due to increased work of the right ventricle. In tricuspid atresia there is left ventricular hypertrophy. The ECG changes of right ventricular hypertrophy include rsR pattern in lead V1, upright T wave in lead V1 after the age of 72 hours, and R Wave in lead V1 of more than 15 mm.

8.9. Which of the following is/are important in assessing ventricular hypertrophy on electrocardiogram?

A   PR interval.
B   T wave morphology.
C   R wave voltage.
D   Frontal plane axis.
E   Heart rate.

8.10. Which of the following statements is/are correct?

A   Tricuspid atresia is the commonest type of cyanotic congenital heart disease.
B   In tetralogy of Fallot the child typically adopts a squatting position after exertion.
C   Notching of the ribs will not be seen in a 6-month-old infant with coarctation of the aorta.
D   The murmur of atrial septal defect is due to flow across the defect.
E   Following surgical correction of vascular ring, stridor will resolve in more than 80% of cases.

8.11. Which of the following statements is/are true of uncomplicated patent ductus arteriosus in a 2-year-old child?

A   It should be ligated.
B   The patient should be given indomethacin.
C   It may present with cyanosis and clubbing.
D   ECG shows right ventricular hypertrophy.
E   X-ray chest shows increase in vascular markings.

8.12. Which of the following is/are true of patent ductus arteriosus?

A   The murmur of a patent ductus arteriosus can be heard in more than 50% of apparently normal babies in the second week of life.
B   If a patent ductus arteriosus is present at 6 months of age, the chances of spontaneous closure are less than 3%.
C   A small patent ductus arteriosus can be complicated by endocarditis.
D   Congestive cardiac failure is a recognized complication.
E   Ligation of the PDA should preferably be deferred until the child is older than 4 years.

8.9. B C D
Ventricular hypertrophy is diagnosed by studying the morphology of T waves in the chest leads, voltage of the R waves and the position of the axis of the heart. PR interval indicates the time taken for the electrical impulse to travel from the SA node to the AV node. The heart rate does not reflect the state of the ventricles.

8.10. B C
Tricuspid atresia is the least common type of cyanotic heart disease. Transposition of the great vessels is the commonest type of cyanotic congenital heart disease at birth. Characteristically children with tetralogy of Fallot assume a squatting position for the relief of dyspnoea due to physical effort but are able to resume physical activity within a few minutes. Notching of the ribs is seen with coarctation of the aorta in later childhood. The murmur of atrial septal defect is due to increased flow of blood across the pulmonary outflow tract and valve. The stridor associated with vascular ring persists after correction in more than 50% of the cases as they have concomitant tracheomalacia as well.

8.11. A E
Ductus arteriosus which does not close by the age of 2 years needs to be ligated as there is a risk of subacute bacterial endocarditis and pulmonary hypertension. In patent ductus arteriosus there is increase in pulmonary blood flow which shows as increase in vascular markings on chest X-ray. Right ventricular hypertrophy, cyanosis and clubbing can occur if the patient develops pulmonary hypertension. In uncomplicated patent ductus arteriosus the ECG shows left ventricular hypertrophy.

8.12. B C D
Physiological closure of the ductus arteriosus occurs within 24 hours of birth in more than 90% of cases and therefore no murmurs are heard. When the ductus arteriosus persists beyond the neonatal period it is due to structural abnormality (deficiency of both the epithelial and muscular layers) which prevents spontaneous closure. Treatment is best carried out between the age of 1–2 years (as spontaneous closure is uncommon after this age) because of the risk of subacute bacterial endarteritis, pulmonary hypertension and congestive cardiac failure.

8.13. Which of the following statements is/are true of coarctation of aorta?
A   Hypertension may be the presenting symptom.
B   The left ventricle is enlarged.
C   The murmur is due to increased blood flow through the aortic valve.
D   The femoral pulse may be of normal amplitude.
E   Subacute bacterial endocarditis prophylaxis is not required after corrective surgery.

8.14. Which of the following are classically found in severe aortic stenosis?
A   Small carotid pulse.
B   Fourth heart sound.
C   Prominent left ventricular impulse.
D   Giant A waves.
E   Radio-femoral delay.

8.15. Which of the following are found in atrial septal defect?
A   A mid-systolic murmur in the pulmonary area.
B   Fixed splitting of the second heart sound.
C   A systolic thrill.
D   Splitting of the first heart sound.
E   A mid-diastolic murmur at the apex.

8.16. Which of the following statements is/are true of atrial septal (septum secundum) defect?
A   The systolic murmur is usually present at birth.
B   The systolic murmur is due to increased flow across pulmonary outflow tract and valve.
C   There is fixed splitting of the second heart sound.
D   The lung fields are plethoric.
E   There is no risk of pulmonary hypertension.

8.13. A B D

In coarctation of the aorta the left ventricle is enlarged because of obstruction to the flow of blood through the narrowed aorta and hypertension because of disturbance of renal blood flow. The femoral pulse may be of normal amplitude though it may be delayed. Prophylaxis for subacute bacterial endocarditis should be continued even after surgery. A short systolic murmur is heard along the left sternal edge in the 3rd and 4th left intercostal spaces. The murmur is transmitted to the back and neck.

8.14. A B C

In severe aortic stenosis the pulse amplitude is low and there is left ventricular enlargement. A prominent fourth heart sound is audible. There is no difference between the radial and femoral pulses and the jugular venous pulse is normal.

8.15. A B E

In atrial septal defect there is an ejection systolic murmur in the pulmonary area due to increased flow across the right ventricular outflow tract, fixed splitting of the second heart sound which is due to constantly increased right ventricular diastolic volume and prolonged ejection time. There is a mid-diastolic murmur at the lower left sternal border due to high blood flow across the tricuspid valve. There are no thrills and the first heart sound is normal.

8.16. B C D

The murmur of atrial septal defect is not present at birth. It is due to increased flow across the pulmonary outflow tract and valve. The fixed splitting is due to constantly increased right ventricular diastolic volume and prolonged ejection time. There is increased blod flow to the lungs which is seen as pulmonary plethora on X-ray. Pulmonary hypertension can result because there is increased blood flow to the lung.

8.17. Which of the following statements is/are true of ventricular septal defects (VSD) in children?
A   Bacterial endocarditis is always a risk, even in heamodynamically insignificant VSDs.
B   In large VSDs a mitral diastolic murmur is indicative of congenital mitral valve pathology.
C   If the VSD is still present at 2 years of age, there is less than 2% chance of spontaneous closure by 10 years of age.
D   A loud pulmonary component of the second sound is reassuring, as it means that a decrease in the shunt from left to right is imminent.
E   VSDs account for about 10% of all congenital cardiac lesions.

8.18. Which of the following is/are associated with Fallot's tetralogy?
A   Cerebral haemorrhage.
B   Squatting.
C   Cyanotic spells.
D   Cerebral abscess.
E   Unsplit second heart sound.

8.19. Which of the following statements is/are characteristic of tetralogy of Fallot?
A   The heart appears enlarged on chest X-ray.
B   Cyanosis is usually present at birth.
C   The pulmonary valve may be normal.
D   The aortic arch is on the right in more than 20% of cases.
E   The aorta is smaller than normal.

8.20. Which of the following statements is/are true of transposition of great arteries?
A   The aorta lies posterior to the pulmonary artery.
B   The aorta receives blood from the left ventricle.
C   Cyanosis usually disappears when 100% oxygen is inspired for 10 minutes.
D   If a large patent ductus arteriosus is discovered at cardiac catheter, urgent arrangements for ligation of the duct must be made.
E   Confirmation of diagnosis is urgent.

8.17. A
Bacterial endocarditis occurs because of the deformity of the ventricular septum and has nothing to do with the size of the defect. The mitral diastolic murmur in ventricular septal defect is due to relative narrowing of the mitral valve and is not due to any pathology. Spontaneous closure of ventricular septal defect can occur as late as 5 years. A loud pulmonary second sound in VSD indicates the onset of pulmonary hypertension. Ventricular septal defect is the most common cardiac malformation and accounts for approximately 25% of congenital heart disease.

8.18. B C D E
Cyanotic spells are a particular problem in tetralogy of Fallot during the first 2 years of life. They are associated with a reduction of an already compromised pulmonary blood flow. The second heart sound is single, it is produced by closure of the aortic valve alone since the pulmonary valve closure is not heard. Characteristically, children assume a squatting position for the relief of breathlessness due to physical effort and the child is usually able to resume physical activity within a few minutes. Cerebral complications such as thrombosis, ischaemia and abscess are recognized complications of tetralogy of Fallot.

8.19. A C D
In tetralogy of Fallot the right ventricle is enlarged. Cyanosis may not be present at birth. The pulmonary obstruction is usually at the right ventricular outflow tract and the pulmonary valve may be normal. The aortic arch is right-sided in 20% of cases. The aorta overrides the ventricular defect and is normal in size.

8.20. E
In transposition the aorta lies anterior and to the right of the pulmonary trunk. It receives blood from the right ventricle. Administration of oxygen does not affect the cyanosis. It is important that the ductus arteriosus remains open as it may be the only communication between the heart and the lungs. Immediate investigation by echocardiogram (and treatment by balloon septostomy) is necessary in order to ensure that blood supply to the lungs is maintained (or adequate mixing of venous and arterial blood is possible). Prostaglandins are indicated if there are signs of closure of the ductus arteriosus before investigations can be undertaken.

8.21. Which of the following congenital cardiac defects present with cyanosis?

A Complete transposition of the great arteries.
B Tricuspid atresia.
C Isolated ventricular septal defect.
D Aortic stenosis.
E Total anomalous pulmonary venous drainage.

8.22. In congenital heart disease, cyanosis

A is distinguished from that of respiratory origin by its failure to diminish on breathing 100% oxygen for 10 minutes.
B requires at least 5 g/100 ml of reduced Hb for recognition.
C causes polycythaemia.
D characteristically causes hyperventilation and respiratory alkalosis.
E requires urgent investigation.

8.23. Which of the following are associated with finger clubbing?

A Aortic coarctation.
B Tricuspid atresia.
C Tetralogy of Fallot.
D Asthma.
E Partial atrioventricular septal defect.

8.24. Which of the following is/are true of acute rheumatic fever?

A Acute rheumatic carditis with heart failure is a generally accepted indication for corticosteroid treatment.
B Mitral stenosis is a major manifestation of acute rheumatic fever.
C The murmur of aortic incompetence is a recognized feature of acute rheumatic carditis.
D Mitral incompetence occurring during acute rheumatic carditis is permanent unless surgically corrected.
E A transient mid-diastolic murmur is characteristic of acute rheumatic carditis.

8.21. A B E
Cyanosis is a presenting symptom of transposition of the great arteries, tricuspid atresia and total anomalous pulmonary venous drainage. In all these conditions there is mixing of the arterial with venous blood which is not the case with aortic stenosis and ventricular septal defect.

8.22. A B C E
Cyanosis of respiratory origin improves following administration of oxygen whereas that due to cardiac disease remains unchanged. Cyanosis is due to the presence of unoxygenated haemoglobin and a minimum of 5 g/100 ml of de-oxygenated haemoglobin is necessary for the naked eye to recognize cyanosis. Cyanosis indicates hypoxia which causes bone marrow hyperplasia resulting in polycythaemia. Patients with cyanotic congenital heart disease need urgent investigations (and treatment) as they may be depending on the ductus arteriosus (which may close up) to maintain adequate oxygenation. Cyanosis in congenital heart disease unless complicated with metabolic acidosis does not cause hyperventilation.

8.23. B C
Clubbing of fingers occurs in cyanotic congenital heart disease (tricuspid atresia, tetralogy of Fallot), suppurative lung disease (bronchiectasis, cystic fibrosis), liver disease or may be congenital.

8.24. A C E
Acute rheumatic fever can result in pancarditis. The mitral and aortic valves are most commonly involved. In acute phase involvement of the mitral valve is manifested as a mid-diastolic murmur which may resolve. Mitral stenosis is a late complication of the involvement of the valve. The lesions of the aortic valve result in aortic incompetence or less commonly, aortic stenosis. Mitral incompetence in the acute phase may resolve spontaneously.

8.25. Which of the following statements is/are true of acute rheumatic fever?
A Initial treatment should include penicillin.
B Fever, polyarthralgia and an elevated ASO titre are sufficient to establish the diagnosis.
C The heart murmur most often heard in acute rheumatic carditis is the murmur of mitral incompetence.
D Rheumatic chorea has a special tendency to occur as an isolated symptom in an otherwise well person.
E After acute rheumatic carditis, prophylaxis with oral penicillin is recommended.

8.26. Prophylaxis with penicillin against subacute bacterial endocarditis in a patient with congenital heart disease is
A inadequate treatment for a child requiring abdominal surgery.
B not necessary in a patient with a very small ventricular septal defect.
C adequate treatment in a patient requiring dental treatment.
D not indicated in a patient who has had his ductus arteriosus ligated and who has no other cardiac lesions.
E indicated if the patient has an upper respiratory tract infection.

8.25.   A C E
The association between streptococcal infections and acute rheumatic fever is well established. Management of acute rheumatic fever includes a course of penicillin to eliminate streptococcal infection. The diagnosis of acute rheumatic fever is based on Jones' criteria which include two major manifestations (carditis, polyarthritis, chorea, erythema marginatum, subcutaneous nodules) or one major and two minor manifestations (fever, arthralgia, previous rheumatic fever or rheumatic heart disease, raised ASO titre, raised ESR, leucocytosis, C-reactive protein, prolonged P–R interval). Mitral valve is the most common valve involved and usually presents with the murmur of mitral incompetence. As the relationship between acute rheumatic carditis and streptococcal infection is well established, appropriate treatment consists of therapeutic dosages of penicillin followed by long-term penicillin prophylaxis. Rheumatic chorea is often accompanied with emotional lability, deterioration in school performance and poor coordination. The affected muscles are weak and the deep tendon reflexes are variable.

8.26.   A C D
For abdominal surgery, prophylaxis against subacute bacterial endocarditis requires gentamicin (for gram-negative organisms of gut) in addition to penicillin. It should be offered to all patients with congenital or acquired heart disease. Penicillin is adequate treatment for the patient requiring dental treatment. It is not indicated for a patient who had his ductus arteriosus ligated and who has an upper respiratory tract infection.

9 Haematology and oncology

9.1. You are asked to see a 5-week-old baby whose birth weight was 1.360 kg. Delivery was normal and his haemoglobin at birth was normal and the baby has fed and gained weight well. However, his haemoglobin is now 9 g. You would expect the anaemia to be due to

A   increase in blood volume.
B   lack of iron intake.
C   normal attrition and non-replacement of red blood cells.
D   increased fragility of red cells.
E   lack of iron absorption.

9.2. Which of the following haematological value/s is/are within normal limits?

A   Haemoglobin of 14 g/100 ml in a 1-month-old boy.
B   White cell count of $12 \times 10^9/1$ with 16% neutrophils in a 6-month-old boy.
C   White cell count of $15 \times 10^9/1$ with 70% lymphocytes in a 6-month-old boy.
D   Haemoglobin F of 2% in a 1-year-old boy.
E   Platelet count of $80 \times 10^9/1$ in a normal full-term infant.

9.3. Fetal haemoglobin

A   has more iron content as compared to adult haemoglobin.
B   has higher oxygen binding capacity.
C   is the sole haemoglobin that can be identified during fetal life.
D   forms the major fraction of total haemoglobin during late infancy.
E   is resistant to alkali denaturation.

9.4. Causes of iron deficiency in a 2-year-old child include

A   consumption of proprietary formulae made from cow's milk.
B   feeding fads.
C   acute glomerulonephritis.
D   coeliac disease.
E   premature birth.

9.1. A C
Premature infants grow very rapidly and increase their blood volume. The bone marrow is unable to put out enough red blood cells to maintain the haemoglobin. Anaemia in premature infants also occurs because of 'physiological hypoplasia' of the marrow. Iron deficiency anaemia of prematurity does not appear till the age of 3–6 months. Though premature infants may contain larger amounts of fetal haemoglobin which may cause slightly increased fragility of the red cells, it does not account for the anaemia. Absorption of iron is normal compared to full-term infants.

9.2. A B C D
The values mentioned in A, B, C and D are normal. The platelet counts are 150 000 to 400 000/cmm.

9.3. B E
Fetal haemoglobin has the same content of iron as adult haemoglobin but has greater affinity for oxygen which shifts the oxygen dissociation curve to the left. Though it is the major form of haemoglobin in fetal life (90% at 28 weeks, 70% at term), adult haemoglobin progressively increases as gestation progresses and very small amounts (less than 2%) of haemoglobin F are present in late infancy. It is resistant to alkali denaturation.

9.4. B D
Iron deficiency does not occur in infants fed on proprietary formulae made from cow's milk as such milks contain iron. In acute glomerulonephritis the blood loss in the urine is very small and therefore iron deficiency does not occur. Iron deficiency anaemia in premature infants usually occurs between the age of 3–6 months. Iron deficiency may result from feeding fads because such foods may not contain iron and with coeliac disease because of poor absorption of iron.

9.5. An 11-month-old child with parents of Greek origin presents with irritability and pallor. He has a haemoglobin level of 7 g/100 ml and hypochromic microcytic blood film. His serum ferritin level is below normal. Which of the following statements is/are correct?

A   He most probably has beta-thalassaemia major.
B   A dietary history is important.
C   Occult bleeding should be excluded.
D   The parents should be tested for evidence of thalassaemia trait if this has not been done before.
E   A low serum ferritin indicates depletion of iron stores.

9.6. An 11-month-old boy presents with pallor. There is no bruising or hepatosplenomegaly. His mother is of Italian and his father is of English origin. His haemoglobin is 3.5 g/100 ml. The blood film shows hypochromic microcytic red cells and the white cells show normal morphology. Which of the following is/are correct?

A   This disease is a sex-linked disorder.
B   A dietary history is very important.
C   Long-term treatment with blood transfusion will be required.
D   A bone marrow examination is indicated.
E   Adequate intake of cereals might have prevented this child's anaemia.

9.7. Megaloblastic anaemia is likely to occur in infants

A   fed on soya formula.
B   fed on goat's milk.
C   undergoing resection of ileum.
D   with gastro-oesophageal reflux.
E   with colostomy for Hirschsprung's disease.

9.8. Which of the following is/are characteristic of haemolytic anaemias?

A   Reticulocytosis.
B   Raised haptoglobin.
C   Raised conjugated bilirubin.
D   Hypochromic erythrocytes.
E   Urobilin in urine.

9.5. B C D E
In the presence of hypochromic microcytic anaemia and low serum ferritin levels the diagnosis is iron deficiency anaemia. In thalassaemia peripheral blood film will show nucleated red blood cells and target cells. Poor iron intake (no solids in the diet) and occult blood loss are the commonest causes of iron deficiency in infants and children. In view of the ethnic background, it is important to ensure that the parents do not have thalassaemia trait. Serum ferritin is the only blood test that allows the evaluation of iron reserves.

9.6. B E
Hypochromic microcytic anaemia occurs due to iron deficiency in which there may be slight splenomegaly and hepatomegaly unlike thalassaemia major in which the liver and spleen are much enlarged and there are target cells and nucleated red blood cells. In an 11-month-old child the most likely cause of iron deficiency is a diet deficient in iron (no solids in the diet). Cereals are a very rich source of iron though some of them are fortified with iron. The infant can be treated with supplemental iron and blood transfusions are not indicated. Leukaemia is an unlikely diagnosis because the morphology of the white cells is normal. Parents' ethnic origin is not relevant in iron deficiency anaemia.

9.7. B C
Megaloblastic anaemia in infants fed on goat's milk is due to deficiency of folic acid. That due to resection of ileum is due to vitamin B_{12} malabsorption. Anaemia due to gastro-oesophageal reflux is due to blood loss leading to iron deficiency. There is no anaemia associated with soya formula or Hirschsprung's disease.

9.8. A E
In haemolytic anaemias, the reticulocyte count is increased, haptoglobin levels are decreased (haptoglobin-haemoglobin complex is excreted), red blood cells are normochromic and unconjugated bilirubin levels are increased. There is increased urobilin but no bile in the urine.

9.9. Which of the following statements is/are true of thalassaemia major?

A   There is a defect in synthesis of haemoglobin A.
B   The condition may be readily recognizable in the newborn by haemoglobin electrophoresis.
C   Abnormalities will usually be found in the blood film of both parents.
D   Spherocytes are characteristically found in the peripheral blood film.
E   It can be diagnosed in utero by amniotic fluid examination.

9.10. Which of the following is/are true of thalassaemia major?

A   Diagnosis can be made at birth by haemoglobin electrophoresis.
B   Fetal haemoglobin levels are elevated at the time of diagnosis.
C   The likelihood of a sibling similarly affected is 1 in 2.
D   Parents are likely to have raised levels of fetal haemoglobin exceeding 20%.
E   Desferrioxamine should not be administered until after the age of 6 years because of toxic effects.

9.11. Which of the following statements is/are true of hereditary spherocytosis (HS)?

A   About 50% of affected infants have moderately severe neonatal jaundice.
B   The diagnosis can be made easily in the newborn period by examination of a blood film.
C   'Crises' during childhood are usually aplastic.
D   Intravascular haemolysis is a common feature.
E   The disorder is usually due to autosomal recessive inheritance.

9.12. Which of the following is/are true of hereditary spherocytosis?

A   It is inherited as an autosomal dominant.
B   The symptoms are relieved by splenectomy.
C   Pigment gallstones occur in over 20% of children before the age of 14 years.
D   Patients with this condition should avoid oxidizing agents such as primaquin, because of the risk of haemolytic crisis.
E   The red cell morphology reverts to normal after splenectomy.

9.9. A C
In thalassaemia major there is impaired synthesis of beta chains of haemoglobin which are required for the synthesis of haemoglobin A. As a result haemoglobin F is formed. As haemoglobin F is normally present in the newborn period, haemoglobin electrophoresis will not establish the diagnosis. Blood of the parents (heterozygotes) shows elevations of haemoglobin A2 (3.5–7%) and haemoglobin F (2–6%). The peripheral blood film shows hypochromia, target cells and nucleated red blood cells. In utero diagnosis is made by sampling fetal blood and analysing haemoglobin chains.

9.10. B
Diagnosis of thalassemia major is made by demonstration of raised levels of fetal haemoglobin which is normally present in the newborn infant. The disease is autosomal recessive which results in an incidence of 1 in 4 in siblings. Haemoglobin F levels in heterozygotes (parents) are usually less than 5% though in some cases may be up to 15%. Haemoglobin A2 levels vary between 3.5 and 7%. Desferrioxamine could be administered at any age though it is usually not commenced till the age of 1 year because of technical problems.

9.11. A
About half the infants with hereditary spherocytosis will develop jaundice severe enough to require phototherapy. In the newborn period ABO incompatibility can present with spherocytes in the peripheral blood film which can be confused with hereditary spherocytosis. Aplastic crisis account for less than 5% of all 'crises'. Usually there is haemolysis and decreased red cell production rather than true aplasia. There is no intravascular haemolysis. The disorder is autosomal dominant.

9.12. A B
Hereditary spherocytosis is autosomal dominant. As the majority of cells are destroyed by the spleen, splenectomy relieves the symptoms. Though gallstones have been reported in children as young as 4–5 years of age, in most cases they occur in late childhood or adolescence. Haemolysis occurs because of the abnormality of the cells and not due to oxidizing agents. Red cell morphology remains unchanged after splenectomy.

9.13. A 4-year-old boy presents with anaemia and dark urine. Urine examination is positive for blood but no red blood cells are seen on microscopy. Which of the following statements is/are correct?

A   Recent dietary history is important.
B   A raised blood pressure would suggest a diagnosis of acute nephritis.
C   The most likely diagnosis is hemolytic-uraemic syndrome.
D   The condition is unlikely to be life threatening.
E   A family history of gallstones or jaundice is important in elucidating the diagnosis.

9.14. Rh-immune globulin prevents Rh isoimmunizaton by

A   neutralizing Rh-immune globulin formed by the Rh-negative mother.
B   coating Rh-positive cells and preventing exposure of the Rh antigen to the maternal immune mechanism.
C   stimulating the mother to produce anti-Rh human globulin which destroys actively produced Rh antibody.
D   competing with RH antigen for albumin binding sites.
E   eliminating RH-positive cells from the maternal circulation.

9.15. An infant or young child whose spleen is removed following traumatic rupture has an increased risk of developing

A   thrombocytopenia.
B   haemolytic anaemia.
C   leukaemia.
D   polycythemia.
E   severe bacterial infection.

9.16. A preponderance of lymphocytes in the differential white cell count is characteristic in

A   infants at birth.
B   infants at 3 months.
C   children aged 10 years.
D   whooping cough.
E   infectious mononucleosis.

147

9.13. A E
The history suggests intravascular haemolysis with haemoglobinuria. Severe haemolysis occurs in G-6-PD deficiency on ingestion of fava beans. A family history of gallstones indicates the presence of a familial haemolytic anaemia. In acute nephritis and haemolytic-uraemic syndrome there are red blood cells seen on microscopy. As the intravascular haemolysis may be accompanied with aplasia it may be life threatening.

9.14. E
Rh-immune globulin eliminates Rh-positive cells from the maternal circulation thereby preventing the mother from being isoimmunized. The RH-immune globulin formed by the RH-negative mother is the same as the administered Rh-immune globulin and therefore it cannot neutralize it or stimulate the production of anti-Rh immune globulin which would destroy the actively produced Rh antibody. The Rh antigen does not bind to albumin to produce antibodies. The Rh-immune globulin does not just coat the Rh-positive cells but actively destroys them thus eliminating them from the maternal circulation.

9.15. E
Removal of the spleen alters host resistance and often results in fatal septicaemia or meningitis. Immediately after splenectomy the platelets are increased and they may be normal later. There is no increase in risk of haemolytic anaemia, leukaemia or polycythemia.

9.16. B D E
At birth infants have lower lymphocyte count. After the first week of life they have relative lymphocytosis before approaching adult proportions at the age of 10 years. There is lymphocytosis in whooping cough and infectious mononucleosis. In the latter condition the lymphocytes are atypical.

9.17. Idiopathic thrombocytopenic purpura in children

A often follows a viral infection.
B typically has a chronic course, with relapses following each remission.
C is characteristically associated with moderate splenomegaly.
D is associated with a reduction of megakaryocytes on bone marrow examination.
E requires splenectomy in more than 20% of cases.

9.18. Platelet transfusion may be indicated in patients with

A haemophilia.
B Henoch–Schönlein purpura.
C aplastic anaemia.
D chronic idiopathic thrombocytopenic purpura.
E lupus erythematosus.

9.19. A boy aged 6 years has a history of severe bruising and petechiae of several days' duration. He is not anaemic. There is no enlargement of liver or spleen. Which of the following statements is/are true of this patient?

A The most likely diagnosis is idiopathic thrombocytopenic purpura.
B Bone marrow examination will show numerous megakaryocytes.
C Complete recovery would be expected in 3–6 weeks' time in more than 80% of cases.
D Bleeding in joints is a likely complication.
E Splenectomy is recommended if the disease is still active after 3–4 months.

9.20. Which of the following statements is/are true of anaphylactoid (Henoch–Schönlein) purpura?

A The platelet count is less than $100 \times 10^9/1$.
B Microscopic haematuria may persist for more than 1 year.
C Intussusception is a recognized complication.
D The arthritis may lead to joint deformity.
E There is evidence to suggest that it is an immune complex disease.

9.17. A
Approximately 60% of patients with idiopathic thrombocytopenic purpura give a history of preceding viral infections. Relapses rarely follow a remission though in a chronic case the problem may persist. There is no splenomegaly and megakaryocytes are either normal or increased. About 90% of children regain normal platelet counts within 9–12 months of onset of disease.

9.18. C
Bleeding in haemophilia is due to factor VIII or factor IX deficiency (coagulation problems), in Henoch–Schönlein purpura it is due to vascular fragility. Platelet transfusion is indicated in bleeding episodes of aplastic anaemia. It is not indicated in chronic idiopathic thrombocytopenic purpura because bleeding episodes are extremely rare. In immune thrombocytopenic purpura due to lupus erythematosus the platelets are rapidly destroyed and are of little benefit to the patient.

9.19. A B C
Tendency to bleed with low platelet count and without hepatosplenomegaly support the diagnosis of idiopathic thrombocytopenic purpura in which there are numerous megakaryocytes in the bone marrow. The majority of these patients recover in 6 weeks' time. There is no bleeding in the joints as the other clotting factors are normal. Splenectomy is indicated only if the disease is severe and fails to respond to corticosteroids and gammaglobulins or if chronic (more than one year).

9.20. B C E
Henoch–Schönlein purpura is the most common form of systemic vasculitis in children which is presumed to be an immune complex disease as immunofluorescense shows mesangial deposits of IgA in association with IgG, C3 and fibrin. The platelet count is normal. The principle manifestations are arthritis or arthralgia which causes no deformity, abdominal pain sometimes accompanied with intussusception, urticarial/purpuric rash involving the buttocks and lower limbs and haematuria which may persist for years. The renal lesion sometimes progresses to chronic renal failure.

9.21. Haemophilia is associated with

A petechiae.
B prolonged skin bleeding time.
C prolonged prothrombin time.
D Factor VIII deficiency.
E haemarthrosis.

9.22. A 5-year-old child receiving maintenance chemotherapy for acute lymphoblastic leukaemia presents with a temperature of 39°C, but no other symptoms. Appropriate immediate measures include

A full blood count.
B blood culture.
C bone marrow aspiration.
D checking respiratory rate.
E lumbar puncture.

9.23. A parent of an 8-year-old child receiving chemotherapy for leukaemia is notified from school that another child has chickenpox. Which of the following is/are necessary in the management of this child?

A Establish whether the leukaemic child has had chickenpox.
B Give a course of acyclovir.
C Establish the proximity of contact in school.
D Establish the timing of contact in school.
E Give pooled gammaglobulin injection.

9.24. Which of the following is/are true about the toxic effects of anticancer drugs?

A Cyclophosphamide may cause cystitis.
B Vincristine causes myopathy.
C Corticosteroids cause a peripheral neuropathy.
D Anthracyclines may be cardiotoxic.
E Methotrexate causes gastrointestinal ulceration.

9.21. D E

Haemophilia is caused by factor VIII and factor IX deficiency. It results in haemarthrosis because of bleeding in the joints which fails to stop. As the platelets are normal, there is no increase in bleeding time or prothrombin time. Petechiae are not a feature of haemophilia.

9.22. A B D

Leukaemic children receiving chemotherapy who develop fever are most likely to have septicaemia or respiratory infections. Diagnosis is made by full blood count which shows leucopenia, blood culture and counting the respiratory rate (chest signs are rarely present). Meningitis is extremely rare and bone marrow aspiration is not indicated.

9.23. C D

Chickenpox is a very serious disease in a leukaemic child and past infection does not prevent the child from reinfection. Acyclovir may be used but is not necessary. It is important to establish the proximity of the contact and to establish the time of contact as it will allow to monitor the incubation period closely. Pooled gammaglobulin is not useful though hyperimmune gammaglobulin is effective when given within 72 hours of exposure.

9.24. A D E

Unexpected side effects of cyclophosphamide are haemorrhagic cystitis and colitis, pulmonary interstitial fibrosis and cardiomyopathy (when given in large doses). Methotrexate causes gastrointestinal ulceration, skin rashes, central nervous system symptoms (aphasia, hemiparesis, motor neuropathy), pneumonitis and hyperglycaemia. Anthracyclines (daunorubicin hydrochloride) cause cardiotoxicity, alopecia and renal failure. Vincristine causes alopecia and peripheral neuropathy but no myopathy. Corticosteroids may cause myopathy but not peripheral neuropathy.

9.25. Acute lymphoblastic leukaemia
A   is the commonest childhood malignancy.
B   is accompanied by splenomegaly in more than half of newly diagnosed children.
C   is excluded if no blast cells are seen in the peripheral blood film.
D   seldom produces intracranial complications.
E   treatment places the child at grave risk from infection by varicella and measles.

9.26. The differential diagnosis in a 3-year-old child with a palpable right abdominal mass includes
A   Wilms' tumour.
B   non-Hodgkin's lymphoma.
C   mesoblastic nephroma.
D   neuroblastoma.
E   hepatoblastoma.

9.27. A boy aged 4 years has a large abdominal mass, X-ray and CT scan of his chest showed multiple round intrapulmonary metastases. Which of the following is/are likely?
A   Neuroblastoma.
B   Wilms' tumour.
C   Non-Hodgkin's lymphoma.
D   Hodgkin's disease.
E   Rhabdomyosarcoma.

9.28. Which of the following statements is/are true of Wilms' tumour?
A   It is the most common malignant tumour of the genitourinary tract of childhood.
B   With current treatment 5-year survival exceeds over 60%.
C   There is an increased incidence of congenital hemihypertrophy in this tumour.
D   Prognosis is less favourable in children under 2 years of age.
E   It presents with haematuria in more than 70% of cases.

153

9.25. A B E
Acute lymphoblastic leukaemia is the commonest childhood malignancy (cerebral malignancy is second). Splenomegaly is a common finding. Treatment consists of chemotherapy which lowers the host immune responses and makes them liable to severe infections with varicella and measles. Blast cells are not seen in the peripheral blood in aleukaemic leukaemia. CNS infiltration is common and particularly so during relapses.

9.26. A B D E
Wilms' tumour arises from the kidneys, neuroblastoma from the adrenal gland and hepatoblastoma from the liver which can all present as a mass on the right side of the abdomen. Mesoblastic nephroma is a congenital tumour and occurs in children under the age of 2 years. Non-Hodgkin's abdominal lymphomas occur most frequently in the ileocaecal region and present as an abdominal mass, intestinal obstruction or intussusception.

9.27. B E
Wilms' tumour and rhabdomyosarcoma are two malignancies that present with abdominal masses and intrapulmonary metastases. In neuroblastoma the metastases are in the orbit, liver and bone marrow. In Hodgkin's disease and non-Hodgkin's lymphoma the lesions occur simultaneously in many lymph nodes.

9.28. A B C
Wilms' tumour accounts for almost all renal neoplasms in childhood. It is often accompanied with other congenital anomalies which include genitourinary anomalies (4.4%), hemihypertrophy (2.9%) and sporadic aniridia (1.1%). Prognosis is better in children diagnosed before the age of 2 years and cure rates of more than 60% have been reported in all stages of Wilms' tumour. Microscopic or macroscopic haematuria occurs in 10–25% of cases.

9.29. Neuroblastoma
A   has a worse prognosis in the first year of life.
B   may be a cause of paraplegia.
C   usually does not respond to cytotoxic drugs.
D   may sometimes be cured by bone marrow transplantation.
E   may be monitored by testing urinary catecholamines.

9.30. Which of the following statements is/are true of neuroblastoma?
A   It commonly presents as an abdominal mass in one or other flank.
B   IVP commonly reveals displacement and compression of the pelvicaly-ceal pattern.
C   It affects mainly children between 5 and 10 years of age.
D   Metastasis to bone is unusual.
E   A specific aid to preoperative diagnosis is measurement of urinary excretion of catecholamines.

9.31. Which of the following statements about retinoblastoma is/are true?
A   Systemic metastases are usually present at diagnosis.
B   It often presents with leukocoria.
C   It may be bilateral.
D   Some cases are dominantly inherited.
E   It has a 50% overall mortality in Western countries in spite of the best available treatment.

9.32. Clinical features of posterior midline cerebellar tumour include
A   visual field defects.
B   truncal ataxia.
C   stiff neck.
D   dystonia.
E   papilloedema.

9.29. B D E
The earlier the age of onset the better is the prognosis in neuroblastoma. Paraplegia is caused because of secondaries in the spine. Treatment of choice is cytotoxic drugs and radiation. In disseminated disease following extensive chemotherapy and radiation bone marrow transplantation may be curative. The level of urinary catecholamines indicates the activity of the tumour.

9.30. A B E
Neuroblastoma is one of the commonest tumours presenting as an intra-abdominal mass other than Wilm' tumour. The tumour displaces the kidney downwards and thereby distorts the pelvicalyceal pattern. The usual age of presentation is less than 5 years. Metastases to bones and bone marrow are common. Catecholamine excretion in urine is increased and is responsible for hypertension.

9.31. B C D
Retinoblastoma spreads by local extension and reaches subarachnoid space and brain. Haematogenous spread is rare. Leukocoria (a creamy-white pupillary reflex) is the first sign other than strabismus and loss of vision. 40% of retinoblastomas are inherited which may be autosomal dominant or a fresh mutation. The tumour may appear in the other eye even years later. Outcome is good if diagnosed and treated early (90% survival).

9.32. B C E
The classical signs of posterior mid-line tumours are ataxia, stiff neck and raised intracranial pressure causing papilloedema. There is no visual field defect (unless there is severe papilloedema) or dystonia.

9.33. Which of the following statements is/are true of brain tumours in childhood?

A   They are a rare form of malignancy.
B   Most tumours are localized below the tentorium.
C   Hemiparesis is a frequent form of presentation.
D   Papilloedema is infrequent.
E   Medulloblastoma is the commonest tumour.

9.33. B E

Next to leukaemias brain tumours are the commonest form of malignancy in childhood. The tumours are most often infratentorial and histologically are medulloblastomas. Raised intracranial pressure causing papilloedema is common and hemiparesis is rare.

10 Nephrology including fluid and electrolytes

10.1. Which of the following statements is/are correct?

A Glomerular filtration rate (corrected for surface area) is higher in babies than in older children.
B Protein in the urine is diagnostic of urinary tract infection.
C Infants are able to concentrate their urine less effectively than older children.
D The urinary protein in nephrotic syndrome is predominantly tubular in origin.
E Significant urinary losses of IgG do not occur in childhood nephrotic syndrome.

10.2. Which of the following statements regarding glomerular function is/are correct?

A Blood urea level in babies correlates well with glomerular filtration rate.
B Serum creatinine levels usually fall with increasing age.
C Glomerular filtration rate (when corrected for surface area) is less than normal adult values in the first month of life.
D Glomerular filtration rate can be measured by renal clearance rate of $^{99}Tc^m$ DTPA.
E Glomerular filtration rate can be determined from a formula utilizing the child's height and plasma creatinine.

10.3. A previously well 1-year-old girl presents with fever (temperature 38.7°C) and irritability of 24 hours' duration. Physical examination is essentially normal with no obvious source of fever identified. The labia are cleaned with normal saline and a bag urine specimen is collected. Results are as follows: 10–100 white cells/cmm, 10–100 red cells/cmm, micro-organisms seen on Gram stain and a mixed growth of >100 000 coliforms/ml is obtained. Which of the following is/are appropriate?

A Start treatment with co-trimoxazole.
B Repeat bag urine collection.
C Arrange urgent micturating cystogram.
D Collect urine by suprapubic aspiration or clean catch.
E Order aspirin to reduce fever.

10.1. C

The rate of glomerular filtration increases until growth ceases towards the end of the second decade of life. Urinary tract infection can only be diagnosed by demonstrating a high colony count in a properly collected specimen of urine. Maximal urinary concentrating capacity of a well newborn infant is 600–700 mosmol/kg water which increases progressively to 1000 mosmol/kg in older children and adults. The urinary protein loss in nephrotic syndrome is mainly glomerular. Albumin and gammaglobulins are lost in urine in children with nephrotic syndrome, the amount of loss depends on the size of the molecule.

10.2. C D E

Blood urea in babies can be increased by increased protein intake. Serum creatinine levels rise with increasing age. The glomerular filtration rate in infants is less than that in adults. It can be measured by renal clearance rate of $^{99}TC^m$ DTPA and it can be calculated from knowing the child's height and plasma creatinine.

10.3. D

The microscopic examination of urine in this girl suggests a diagnosis of urinary tract infection though the specimen for culture suggests contamination of the specimen. To make a definitive diagnosis a further specimen of urine needs to be examined. In order to ensure there is no contamination it should be obtained by clean catch or suprapubic aspiration. Treatment with co-trimoxazole is not justified without making a definitive diagnosis. A further examination of bag urine may be contaminated again and thus delay treatment. Aspirin is not recommended for treatment of fever in children because it has been implicated in causation of Reye's syndrome.

10.4. A 2-week-old boy has developed a fever (temperature 38.8°C) and is lethargic. He is noted to be mildly jaundiced. Examination of bag specimen of urine shows on microscopy: red cells <10/ml, white cells 10–100/ml, organisms seen and culture of urine showed: 10 000–100 000 coliform organisms/ml, sensitive to all antibiotics tested. Which of the following statements is/are correct?

A   Treatment with an appropriate antibiotic should be commenced immediately.

B   Treatment should be withheld until a specimen of urine is obtained by urethral catheterization.

C   Treatment should be withheld until a specimen of urine is obtained by suprapubic bladder aspiration.

D   This baby's jaundice is most likely related to urinary tract infection.

E   Urinary infection at this age is more common in boys than in girls.

10.5. The bacterial count in urine from a patient with urinary tract infection may be falsely low in which of the following circumstances?

A   As a result of contamination of the specimen with antiseptic.

B   In complete ureteric obstruction.

C   When the urine specific gravity is less than 1.003.

D   During prolonged periods of fever.

E   When the specimen is an early morning collection.

10.6. Which of the following statements is/are true of urinary tract infection?

A   Presence of albumin in the urine establishes the diagnosis.

B   The presence of blood in the urine excludes the diagnosis.

C   The presence of white blood cells in the urine does not establish the diagnosis.

D   Jaundice may be a presenting symptom in the newborn.

E   Single dose therapy is not recommended for infants.

10.7. Which of the following statements is/are true of vesicoureteric reflux?

A   Young siblings of children with vesicoureteric reflux should be screened.

B   Incidence increases with increasing age.

C   A normal renal ultrasound appearance in a child of 2 years rules out the possibility of vesicoureteric reflux.

D   Renal ultrasonography is the most sensitive imaging modality in the detection of renal scarring (reflux nephropathy).

E   Amoxicillin is an appropriate antibiotic for long-term prophylaxis for urinary infection in children with vesicoureteric reflux.

10.4. C D E
Microscopic examination of the urine in this child suggests urinary tract infection though the urine specimen for culture does not completely support the diagnosis. Antibiotic treatment should not commence until a diagnosis has been established. As the infant is unwell, it is important to obtain a suitable specimen of urine urgently. This is best achieved by suprapubic bladder aspiration. In newborn infants there is male sex predilection for urinary tract infection. In this age group jaundice may be the presenting symptom.

10.5. A B C
Antiseptics used to clean the vulva may inhibit the growth of organisms. In complete ureteric obstruction the organisms from the obstructed ureter may not be passed in the urine. Dilute urine will have a smaller number of organisms per ml than concentrated urine (found in early morning specimen and fevers).

10.6. C D E
The diagnosis of urinary tract infection can only be established by culture of the urine though it may be suspected if white blood cells are seen in urine on microscopy. The presence or absence of albumin and blood are of no significance in urinary tract infection. In newborn infants urinary tract infection causes conjugated hyperbilirubinaemia. Though single dose therapy has been shown to be efficacious in adults, it has not been demonstrated to be effective in infants.

10.7. A
Familial incidence of vesicoureteric reflux is approximately 10%. Vesicoureteric reflux is uncommon after the age of 5 years. The only definite way of diagnosing vesicoureteric reflux is by a micturating cystourethrogram. DMSA scan is a more sensitive method of diagnosing renal scarring than renal ultrasonography. Trimethoprim with sulphamethoxazole (Bactrim) is the drug of choice for long-term prophylaxis for urinary tract infection in children with vesicoureteric reflux. The organisms develop resistance to amoxycillin very rapidly.

10.8 Which of the following statements is/are true of vesicoureteric reflux and reflux nephropathy?

A   Vesicoureteric reflux is best diagnosed by intravenous urography or renal ultrasound.

B   Vesicoureteric reflux is found in more than 50% of all children presenting with urinary infection.

C   The incidence of vesicoureteric reflux decreases with increasing age.

D   Siblings of patients with vesicoureteric reflux are more likely to have vesicoureteric reflux than the general population.

E   Reflux nephropathy only leads to hypertension in the presence of renal failure.

10.9. Which of the following statements is/are true of post-streptococcal glomerulonephritis?

A   Post-streptococcal glomerulonephritis is the commonest cause of chronic renal failure in children.

B   The most serious problem is hypertensive encephalopathy.

C   ASO titre is the most useful marker of streptococcal infection.

D   Life-long penicillin prophylaxis is recommended.

E   Abnormalities of serum complement usually persist for longer than 3 months.

10.10. Post-streptococcal acute glomerulonephritis is usually associated with

A   rise in ASO titre.

B   fall in C3 complement.

C   rise in serum IgA levels.

D   hypoalbuminaemia.

E   granular tubular casts in urine.

10.11. A child of 5 years presents with fits and coma. Apart from a sore throat the week before his previous health has been satisfactory. There is slight facial and peripheral oedema. Examination of the fundi shows bilateral papilloedema. Fine crepitations are heard throughout the lung fields. Blood pressure is 200/120 mmHg. The urine is rusty in colour and stix testing for blood and protein is positive. Serum urea is 25 mmol/l and electrolytes are normal. Haemoglobin is 8.5 g/dl and haematocrit is 0.25. Which of the following statements is/are correct?

A   Fits and coma are due to the elevated blood urea.

B   Anaemia is due to blood loss.

C   Crepitations are due to heart failure.

D   Urgent treatment with parenteral hypotensives is indicated.

E   Urgent treatment with steroids is indicated.

10.8   C D

Vesicoureteric reflux can only be diagnosed by a micturating cystourethrogram. Its incidence decreases with increasing age and therefore it would not account for more than 50% of all children presenting with urinary tract infection. 10% of siblings of patients with vesicoureteric reflux are likely to have the same problem. Reflux nephropathy is the commonest cause of hypertension in children with or without renal failure.

10.9.   B C

Less than 5% of children with post-streptococcal glomerulonephritis will develop chronic renal failure. Reflux nephropathy is the commonest cause of chronic renal failure in children. Complications of acute glomerular nephritis include renal failure, cardiac failure with or without hypertension and hypertensive encephalopathy (most serious). Of the many markers of streptococcal infection, ASO titre is the most accurate. Life-long penicillin prophylaxis is not recommended as second attacks of acute glomerulonephritis are rare. Serum complement levels are low only during the acute phase of the disease.

10.10.   A B

In post-streptococcal acute glomerulonephritis there is a rise in ASO titre because of preceding streptococcal infection. There is a fall in C3 fraction of complement because of the formation of antigen/antibody complex which is deposited on the glomeruli. Serum IgA and albumin levels are within normal limits. Urine shows granular casts.

10.11.   C D

History of preceding sore throat (presumably streptococcal), peripheral oedema, papilloedema accompanied with hypertension suggest a diagnosis of post-streptococcal glomerulonephritis complicated with hypertensive encephalopathy. Hypertension and cerebral oedema rather than raised blood urea are the cause of the fits. Anaemia in acute glomerulonephritis is due to increase in plasma volume. Patients with acute glomerulonephritis can develop heart failure with or without hypertension. Hypertensive encephalopathy in acute glomerular nephritis can be fatal. The treatment aims to lower the blood pressure. Steroids are of no benefit.

10.12. Which of the following statements is/are true of minimal change nephrotic syndrome in childhood?

A   Proteinuria clears after an adequate course of corticosteroids in at least 75% of cases.

B   Cyclophosphamide is used to induce prolonged remissions in children with frequent relapses.

C   Serum IgG is decreased during relapses.

D   Oedema is routinely treated with oral diuretics.

E   Persistent hypertension would be an unexpected finding.

10.13. A 2-year-old boy presents with generalized swelling which has developed over the preceding week. His urine output has diminished considerably during this period. Physical examination reveals generalized pitting oedema. Blood pressure is 100/75 mmHg. Urine contains protein + + +, hyaline casts +, no RBC or WBC. He is likely to have

A   raised blood urea.

B   increased susceptibility to pneumococcal infection.

C   an increase in plasma volume.

D   selective proteinuria.

E   low levels of serum complement.

10.14. Pneumococcal peritonitis is a known complication of

A   minimal lesion nephrotic syndrome.

B   mesenteric adenitis.

C   acute appendicitis.

D   benign recurrent haematuria.

E   chronic hereditary nephritis (Alport syndrome).

10.15. Which of the following features indicate a poor prognosis in children with nephrotic syndrome?

A   Onset before 1 year of age.

B   Hypertension.

C   Haematuria.

D   Selective proteinuria.

E   Severity of oedema.

10.12. A B C E

In nephrotic syndrome proteinuria clears within a period of 2 weeks in more than 75% of cases. Patients with frequent relapses will respond to treatment with cyclophosphamide. The fall in serum IgG is partly due to loss in the urine and partly to increased catabolism and decreased formation by the liver. Hypertension is unusual. Diuretics are not indicated and may be dangerous because of the decreased plasma volume.

10.13. B D

The history suggests a diagnosis of nephrotic syndrome in which the blood urea is normal or low, serum complement is normal and plasma volume is decreased. There is increased tendency to pneumococcal infections because of low IgG levels. The urine shows selective proteinuria (i.e. larger amounts of low molecular fractions rather than high molecular fractions).

10.14. A

The association of pneumococcal peritonitis with nephrotic syndrome is well recognized and is thought to be due to the low levels of IgG and accompanying ascites. There is no association between pneumococcal peritonitis and benign recurrent haematuria or chronic hereditary nephritis. In mesenteric adenitis the infection is viral and in acute appendicitis the organisms belong to the gut flora (*E. coli* or *Strep. faecalis*).

10.15. A B C

In infants nephrotic syndrome is resistant to treatment and relapses frequently. Hypertension and haematuria in nephrotic syndrome indicate that the renal pathology is other than 'minimal change'. The severity of oedema bears no relationship to the prognosis. Selective proteinuria would indicate a good prognosis.

10.16. A 6-year-old boy has transient macroscopic haematuria at the time of an upper respiratory tract infection. He has a past history of haematuria during two similar infections 6 and 10 months earlier. Which of the following statements is/are likely to be true?

A Renal histology would reveal a focal and/or segmental proliferative glomerulonephritis in about 50% of such cases.
B Serum IgA levels are likely to be elevated.
C The serum level of the 3rd component of complement would be normal.
D Progressive impairment of renal function characteristically occurs with each episode of haematuria.
E The antistreptolysin O titre often does not rise after an episode of haematuria.

10.17. Which of the following statements concerning chronic renal failure in childhood is/are true?

A It is due to glomerulonephritis in more than 50% of cases.
B Growth is generally retarded.
C Anaemia is usually unresponsive to iron, folic acid and Vitamin B_{12}.
D Normal urinalysis is inconsistent with the diagnosis.
E Renal transplant rejection is more frequent in children than in adults aged 20–40 years.

10.18. Chronic renal failure is seen in association with, or as a sequel to

A Henoch-Schönlein purpura.
B urinary tract infection.
C vesicoureteric reflux.
D idiopathic thrombocytopenic purpura.
E Wilms' tumour.

10.19. Which of the following statements is/are true?

A The percentage of intracellular fluid in the fetus decreases with increasing gestational age.
B The extracellular fluid volume constitutes 20–25% of body weight in the older child.
C The infant of the diabetic mother has an increased percentage of extracellular fluid volume.
D The percentage of extracellular fluid volume tends to decrease with age.
E Total body water represents a smaller percentage of body weight in an obese than in a normal person.

10.16. A C E
Recurrent haematuria in a male child associated with respiratory tract infections supports a diagnosis of IgA nephropathy in which there are focal and/or segmented proliferative changes in the glomeruli. Serum levels of C3 fraction of complement, IgA and streptolysin titre are normal. The condition does not lead to significant kidney damage in most patients.

10.17. B C
Chronic renal failure is characterized by growth failure and anaemia. The latter is due to marrow hypoplasia. Most cases of chronic renal failure in children are due to reflux nephropathy which are followed as a close second by congenital malformations. Urine analysis may show no albumin or red blood cells but specific gravity may be low in end-stage renal disease. Rejection of renal transplant is no more frequent in children than in adults.

10.18. A B C
Henoch–Schönlein purpura, urinary tract infection and vesicoureteric reflux can all cause chronic renal failure. Idiopathic thrombocytopenic purpura does not affect the kidney. Wilms' tumour will either be cured or the child will die due to malignancy before developing renal failure.

10.19. B D E
In the fetus extracellular fluid volume is larger than the intracellular space but the ratio of extracellular fluid to intracellular fluid falls to the adult level by 9 months of postnatal age. In the older child the volume of extracellular fluid is 20–25% of body weight compared to 40% at birth. The extracellular fluid volume is contracted in infants of diabetic mothers. Since fat is low in water content, total body water represents a smaller percentage of body weight in an obese than in a normal person.

10.20. Total body water
A   forms a smaller percentage of body weight in obese as compared to lean children.
B   acounts for approximately 75% of body weight in a term infant.
C   is equally distributed in intracellular and extracellular fluid compartments at 6 months of age.
D   accounts for 40% of infant's weight at 1 year of age.
E   represents increased proportion of body weight in marasmic children.

10.21. Which of the following is/are recognized complications of hypernatraemic dehydration?
A   Fits.
B   Cardiac arrhythmias.
C   Brain damage.
D   Hypertension.
E   Polyuria.

10.22. In hypernatraemic dehydration complicating gastroenteritis
A   there is no potassium loss.
B   there is no sodium loss.
C   intracellular water is preserved.
D   isotonic fluids are required for intravenous rehydration.
E   there is a risk of seizures.

10.23. Potassium
A   is the main intracellular cation of the body.
B   depletion commonly causes diarrhoea.
C   is mainly reabsorbed in the proximal tubule.
D   is mainly excreted in stool.
E   serum levels are sensitive to small changes in total body potassium.

10.20. A B E
Fat is lower in water content, therefore total body water represents a smaller percentage of body weight in an obese than in a normal person. Percentage of body water decreases from conception to adulthood. It is approximately 75% at birth and 60% at the age of 1 year. At 6 months 25% of the body-weight is composed of extracellular fluid and 45% of intracellular fluid. In marasmic children the lean bodyweight is increased in proportion to fat which accounts for increased total body water.

10.21. A C
Hypernatraemic dehydration causes fits during rehydration therapy as a result of brain swelling. Cerebral palsy results because of sagittal sinus thrombosis. Cardiac arrhythmias, hypertension and polyuria are not seen.

10.22. D E
In hypernatraemic dehydration there is loss of electrolytes and water but the water loss is greater. Because of the hypernatraemia intracellular water moves from the cells to the extracellular compartment. It is important to administer isotonic fluids in order to prevent rapid movement of the water back into the cells which may result in cerebral oedema and seizures.

10.23. A C
Intracellular concentrations of potassium approximate 150 mmol/l. Along the length of the proximal renal tubule potassium concentration remains constant indicating that it is reabsorbed in similar proportions to the water, with 60% or more of the filtered potassium being absorbed. Though diarrhoea may cause potassium depletion, potassium depletion causes ileus. Very small amounts of potassium are normally excreted in the stool as most of it is reabsorbed in the gut. As the vast majority of total body potassium is in the intracellular fluid, serum levels are not sensitive to small changes in total body potassium.

10.24. Acute deficiency of potassium may produce
A   tall peaked T waves in the ECG.
B   muscle weakness.
C   ileus.
D   nystagmus.
E   abdominal distension.

10.25. Hypokalaemia is likely to occur with
A   diarrhoea.
B   urinary tract infection.
C   infants of diabetic mothers.
D   infantila pyloric stenosis.
E   neonatal asphyxia.

10.26. Metabolic acidosis is seen in children under which of the following circumstances?
A   Chronic asthma.
B   Hypertrophic pyloric stenosis.
C   Diabetes mellitus.
D   Gastroenteritis.
E   Prolonged fasting.

10.27. Alkalosis may be a problem in
A   infantile gastroenteritis.
B   neonatal duodenal obstruction.
C   hyaline membrane disease.
D   pyloric stenosis.
E   starvation.

10.24. B C E
Hypokalaemia produces functional alterations in muscle which results in lower T wave in ECG, muscle paralysis and ileus which would cause abdominal distension. There is no nystagmus.

10.25. A D
As gastrointestinal fluids contain large quantities of potassium, their loss in diarrhoea and infantile pyloric stenosis results in hypokalaemia. In urinary tract infection there may be hyperkalaemia secondary to renal failure. In neonatal asphyxia potassium leaks out of the cells resulting in hyperkalaemia. There is no disturbance of serum potassium in infants of diabetic mothers.

10.26. C D E
Chronic asthma results in respiratory acidosis as a result of carbon dioxide retention. In hypertrophic pyloric stenosis loss of chloride and hydrogen ions leads to metabolic alkalosis. In diabetes mellitus and prolonged fasting there is increase in ketone bodies resulting in metabolic acidosis. In gastroenteritis there is loss of bicarbonate in the stools resulting in metabolic acidosis.

10.27. B D
Infantile gastroenteritis results in metabolic acidosis due to loss of bicarbonate. Neonatal duodenal obstruction and pyloric stenosis result in alkalosis because of loss of gastric acid juice. Hyaline membrane disease results in a mixed respiratory (raised carbon dioxide tension) and metabolic (anaerobic metabolism) acidosis.

10.28 Which of the following statements is/are true of oral rehydrating fluids?

A   Glucose is essential because it aids in the absorption of electrolytes and water.
B   They contain glucose to supply the full caloric needs of the infant.
C   The sodium and chloride content of the solution is that of normal saline.
D   Sucrose may be substituted for glucose in the solution.
E   The infant may continue breastfeeding while receiving oral rehydration fluid.

10.29. A 1-year-old infant has diarrhoea and vomiting for 3 days. The infant's temperature is 39°C and he is very irritable. There is very little urine being passed but there are no other signs of dehydration. Mother says that she has been feeding full-strength skimmed milk since the commencement of the illness. Which of the following statements is/are correct?

A   Hypernatraemia is likely to be found.
B   The infant should be given 300 ml of 5% dextrose rapidly.
C   The infant is at risk of developing cerebral palsy.
D   Dehydration should be corrected over 48 hours.
E   The infant is not dehydrated.

10.28. A D E

There is active reabsorption of water and electrolytes during the transfer of glucose across the cell membrane. The calories supplied by the glucose in the solution are inadequate. The sodium and chloride content is one-third to one-half normal saline depending on the type of oral rehydrating solution. Sucrose is readily digested even in severe gastroenteritis and can be used as a substitute in oral rehydrating solution. Breastfeeding should be allowed in breastfed infants and water ad lib should be offered to other infants.

10.29. A C D

The presence of diarrhoea, vomiting and scanty urine indicates that the patient is dehydrated. Full-strength skimmed milk is high in electrolytes which will result in hypernatraemia. In such infants the dehydration should be corrected slowly by administration of fluids containing normal or half-normal saline as rapid fluid administration will result in cerebral oedema.

11 Endocrinology and gonads

11.1. Growth hormone secretion in normal individuals is stimulated by which of the following?
A Exercise.
B Hydrocortisone.
C Arginine infusion.
D Insulin-induced hypoglycaemia.
E Sleep.

11.2. Output of growth hormone can be reduced by
A psychosocial deprivation.
B hypoglycaemia.
C exercise.
D sleep.
E malnutrition.

11.3. Congenital hypothyroidism
A is less common than phenylketonuria.
B is reliably detected by biochemical investigation in the first week of life.
C is reliably detected by clinical examination in the first week of life.
D is commonly associated with other endocrine deficiencies.
E causes delay in bone maturation.

11.4. Which of the following is/are likely to be associated with juvenile hypothyroidism presenting at the age of 8 years?
A Ectopic thyroid.
B Athyreosis.
C Obesity.
D Constipation.
E Malformed epiphyses.

11.1. A C D E
Growth hormone secretion is stimulated by sleep, exercise, arginine infusion and hypoglycaemia. Hydrocortisone increases blood glucose and therefore does not stimulate growth hormone secretion.

11.2. A E
Growth hormone production is reduced in psychosocial deprivation and malnutrition but this is not a constant feature in these conditions. Growth hormone production is increased in hypoglycaemia, exercise and sleep.

11.3. B E
The incidence of congenital hypothyroidism is 1 in 4000 compared to that of phenylketonuria which is 1 in 14 000. Careful evaluation of TSH and T4 will establish the diagnosis. There are few reliable physical signs in the first week of life. Usually congenital hypothyroidism is an isolated defect. Bone age is delayed.

11.4. D E
Constipation and malformed epiphyses are classical physical findings in juvenile hypothyroidism. The thyroid gland is always present and is usually not ectopic. Obesity is uncommon.

11.5. Guide(s) to the diagnosis of hypothyroidism in the newborn is/are

A   hypothermia.
B   prolonged hyperbilirubinaemia in the neonatal period.
C   radiographic signs of delay in osseous development.
D   low birth weight for period of gestation.
E   hyperglycaemia.

11.6. A 14-year-old girl has a smooth, non-tender goitre without any other symptoms. Investigations show T4 87 ng/l (normal 85–160), TSH 11 ng/l (normal 2–3.5) and antimicrosomal antibody titre 1/12 500 (normal less than 1/100). Which of the following statements is/are correct?

A   She has compensated hypothyroidism.
B   This presentation of thyroid disease is rare in teenage children.
C   Spontaneous remission of this condition has been observed.
D   Other endocrine abnormalities may also be found.
E   The most likely diagnosis is Grave's disease.

11.7. Enlargement of the thyroid gland may be produced by

A   a deficient intake of iodine.
B   craniopharyngioma.
C   growth hormone.
D   pregnancy.
E   autoimmune disease.

11.8. Which of the following statements is/are true?

A   Propylthiouracil crosses the placenta.
B   Long-acting thyroid stimulating hormone (LATS) crosses the placenta.
C   In untreated hypothyroid children, the legs are disproportionately shorter than the head and trunk.
D   Neonatal hypothyroidism may present as persistent jaundice.
E   Early diagnosis and treatment of congenital hypothyroidism results in normal mental development in most cases.

11.5.   A B C
Hypothyroidism may present with hypothermia at any age group but particularly in the newborn period. The other symptom in the neonatal period is prolonged hyperbilirubinaemia but the levels of bilirubin are not very high. X-rays show delay in bone age and epiphyseal dysgenesis. Newborn infants are normal or large for gestation. Infants with hypothyroidism may present with hypoglycaemia but not hyperglycaemia.

11.6.   A C D
A raised TSH level in the presence of low normal T4 levels supports a diagnosis of compensated hypothyroidism which is most commonly due to Hashimoto thyroiditis in teenage girls. The diagnosis is confirmed by the presence of thyroid antibodies. It has been observed to resolve spontaneously. Clinical manifestations include goitre (which may be euthyroid, hypothyroid or thyrotoxic), other endocrine abnormalities (diabetes mellitus, adrenal insufficiency, hypoparathyroidism) due to auto-antibodies and less commonly pernicious anaemia and thrombocytopenia.

11.7.   A D E
Lack of iodine causes hypertrophy of the acinar tissue and enlargement of the thyroid gland. Craniopharyngioma rarely has any effect on the thyroid gland but may result in decreased TSH production and therefore atrophy of the thyroid gland. Growth hormone does not have any effect on the thyroid gland. Lymphocytic thyroiditis which is an autoimmune disease is the commonest cause of goitre in childhood. There is increase in size of thyroid gland during pregnancy.

11.8.   A B C D E
Propylthiouracil crosses the placenta and may cause congenital hypothyroidism. LATS crosses the placenta and causes severe hyperthyroidism in newborn infants (even though the mother may not have any signs of hyperthyroidism). The legs are shorter in untreated hypothyroid children because of epiphyseal dysgenesis. In neonatal hypothyroidism the jaundice is prolonged but the serum bilirubin is not very high. Recent studies have shown that early treatment of congenital hypothyroidism results in normal development in most but not in all cases.

11.9. Which of the following statements is/are true of the thyroid-stimulating hormone (TSH) level in capillary blood of newborn infants?
A Levels are elevated in congenital hypothyroidism.
B It will detect pituitary hypothyroidism.
C It measures TSH produced by the infant.
D It is suitable for mass screening.
E It is increased in the presence of maternal hypopituitarism.

11.10. Recognized complications of long-term therapy with prednisolone in childhood include
A growth retardation.
B postural hypotension.
C exacerbation of fungal infection.
D proximal myopathy.
E peripheral neuropathy.

11.11. Congenital adrenal hyperplasia
A is associated with high plasma ACTH levels.
B is a common cause of ambiguous genitalia in the newborn.
C may be associated with salt losing.
D is associated with high plasma cortisol levels.
E in males may be associated with infertility.

11.12. Which of the following statements is/are true?
A Congenital adrenal hyperplasia may present as masculinization of a female newborn.
B In congenital adrenal hyperplasia there is often a salt-losing state.
C In testicular feminization syndrome the gonads secrete testosterone, but there is a failure of end organ response.
D Growth hormone deficiency results in disproportionate shortening of the lower limbs.
E In diabetes insipidus, the urine osmolality is relatively increased, while the serum osmolality is relatively decreased.

11.9. A C D

Capillary blood of the newborn shows elevated levels of TSH in congenital hypothyroidism but low levels in pituitary hypothyroidism. TSH does not cross the placenta. It is suitable for mass screening of hypothyroidism other than that due to pituitary disease. Maternal hypopituitarism does not have any effect on the TSH of newborn infants.

11.10. A C D

Corticosteroids cause growth retardation, hypertension, predisposition to infection and myopathy in children.

11.11. A C E

In congenital adrenal hyperplasia the plasma ACTH levels are high. The plasma cortisol levels are normal or low. It should be considered in the differential diagnosis of ambiguous genitalia in the newborn and may occasionally present with hypotension in which case the electrolytes show a low serum sodium (due to salt loss in the urine) and hyperkalaemia. The high androgens may inhibit pituitary secretion of FSH which results in infertility.

11.12. A B C

In newborn female infants the masculinization is due to blockage of the pathway to the formation of hydrocortisone which results in the increased formation of androgens. The salt-losing state is not present in all cases. In testicular feminization syndrome phenotypically the patient is a female though the gonads are testes and there is no uterus. The testes produce testosterone which suggests that there is failure of end organ response. Growth hormone deficiency does not cause any changes in body proportions. In diabetes insipidus, the kidney is unable to concentrate the urine as a result of which there is a decrease in urinary osmolarity and an increase in serum osmolarity.

11.13. A female infant is born with virilization of the external genitalia. Urine examination shows elevation of total 17-hydroxysteroids, 17-ketosteroids and pregnenetriol. Which of the following statements is/are true?

A   Congenital adrenal hyperplasia is the most likely diagnosis.
B   The baby would have normal internal genitalia.
C   The mother has been treated with progestogens.
D   A salt-losing tendency may be present in this infant.
E   The baby will show retardation in bone age.

11.14. Which of the following is/are true of diabetes mellitus with onset in the first decade?

A   It usually occurs in obese children.
B   There is an increase in insulin requirements at puberty.
C   Less insulin is required when appetite is reduced due to acute infections.
D   It should not be treated with oral hypoglycaemic agents.
E   Competitive games should be avoided.

11.15. Which of the following statements is/are true about diabetes mellitus in childhood?

A   It is often treated with oral hypoglycaemic agents.
B   It is a frequent cause of adult blindness.
C   It may present with acute abdominal pain.
D   The concordance rate among monozygotic twins is about 50%.
E   There is good correlation between blood and urine sugar levels.

11.16. Which of the following statement(s) is/are true of diabetes mellitus?

A   Both types of diabetes can occur at any age.
B   Insulin is administered by intramuscular injection.
C   Insulin requirements are usually increased in a patient (whether eating or not) with severe intercurrent illness.
D   Neonatal diabetes mellitus is usually transitory.
E   Congenital rubella is a recognized cause.

11.13. A B D

The clinical presentation and laboratory findings support the diagnosis of adrenal hyperplasia which may have a salt-losing tendency. Bone age is increased because of the androgens which have no effect on internal genitalia of female infants. Progestogens may cause masculinization and increase in pregnenetriol in the urine but there is no elevation of 17-hydroxysteroids and 17-ketosteroids.

11.14. B D

Juvenile diabetes has no relationship to obesity. Insulin requirements increase at puberty. Acute infections increase the requirements of insulin. Juvenile diabetes should not be treated with oral hypoglycaemic agents as there is an absolute lack of insulin production by the pancreas. No restrictions should be placed on activity when the child is well-controlled.

11.15. B C D

As there is an absolute deficiency of insulin in juvenile diabetes mellitus it should not be treated with oral hypoglycaemic agents. Juvenile diabetes mellitus leads to diabetic retinopathy and blindness in adults. Diabetic ketoacidosis is a recognized cause of acute abdominal pain. Though heredity has been implicated in type 1 diabetes mellitus, environmental factors (including autoimmunity) are important as even in monozygotic twins, the concordance rate is only 50%. The blood and urine sugar levels do not correlate well.

11.16. A C D E

Though type 1 diabetes occurs in young patients and type 2 diabetes occurs after the age of 40 years, either type of diabetes can occur at any age. Insulin is administered subcutaneously. If given intramuscularly it will cause necrosis. In severe intercurrent infections the insulin requirements are increased because of increased metabolic rate. The majority of cases of neonatal diabetes mellitus are transitory though some of these patients may develop diabetes later on in life. Congenital rubella results in diabetes mellitus as a result of pancreatitis by the rubella virus.

11.17. A 4-year-old boy presents with drowsiness, hyperpnoea and vomiting. He has been unwell for several days. Acetone can be smelt on his breath and the urine contains sugar in large quantities. Other clinical signs and symptoms associated with this disorder include
A   antecedent increase in thirst.
B   antecedent weight loss.
C   moderate to severe dehydration.
D   severe abdominal pain.
E   Kussmaul breathing (deep sighing respiration).

11.18. A young boy, known to be a diabetic taking insulin, is found unconscious at 11.00 a.m. His mother reports that he went off to school quite well about 8.00 a.m. that morning. You would expect to find
A   hyperventilation.
B   blood glucose below 3.0 mmol/l.
C   ketone bodies in the urine.
D   a good response to injected glucagon.
E   sweating.

11.19. In which of the following may glucose appear in the urine?
A   Fanconi's syndrome.
B   Congenital adrenal hyperplasia.
C   Cerebral haemorrhage.
D   Galactosaemia.
E   Salicylate intoxication.

11.20. Low blood glucose is likely to be found in
A   low birth weight for gestation infants.
B   Cushing's syndrome.
C   glycogen storage disease of the liver.
D   galactosaemia.
E   adrenocortical insufficiency.

11.17.   A B C D E

The stem suggests a diagnosis of juvenile diabetes mellitus. All the distractors are symptoms which may be found in this condition.

11.18.   B D E

The history supports a diagnosis of insulin-induced hypoglycaemia. Hyperventilation which is due to acidosis is a feature of diabetic ketosis. With hypoglycaemia, patients do not have hyperventilation, their blood glucose is low and sweating is a common symptom. Usually there are no ketone bodies in the urine. As their glycogen reserves are high, glucagon will increase their blood glucose.

11.19.   A C E

In Fanconi's syndrome there is glycosuria and aminoaciduria. Cerebral haemorrhage and salicylate intoxication cause hyperglycaemia leading to glycosuria. There is no glycosuria with congenital adrenal hyperplasia. In galactosaemia urine contains reducing substances (galactose) but no glucose.

11.20.   A C D E

The low blood sugar in low birth weight for gestation infants is due to low glycogen reserve, in glycogen storage disease of the liver because of inability to mobilize the glucogen, in galactosaemia due to liver failure as a result of damage to the liver and failure of galactose to enter the metabolic pathway and in adrenocortical insufficiency due to low cortisone levels. In Cushing's syndrome there is hyperglycaemia.

11.21. Which of the following statements is/are true of inappropriate ADH?
A   The serum sodium concentration is low.
B   Urinary output is diminished.
C   Fluid intake should be restricted.
D   Hypertonic saline solution is the treatment of choice.
E   Urinary sodium concentration is low.

11.22. Which of the following statements is/are true?
A   The prepuce cannot be gently retracted in more than 20% of boys by the age of 1 year.
B   If circumcision is desired by the parents, the optimum age for the operation is one week.
C   Circumcision before the child is out of nappies increases the risk of meatal ulcer.
D   If the prepuce cannot be retracted by the age of 5 years, the child needs circumcision.
E   There is no medical indication for circumcision in the newborn infant.

11.23. Which of the following statements is/are true of penile hypospadias?
A   The chordee is often the major functional disability.
B   The urethral meatus is often very narrow.
C   Urethral sphincter is often deficient.
D   Impotence is present in more than 20% of cases.
E   Neonatal circumcision is absolutely contraindicated.

11.24. Posterior urethral valves
A   occur only in males.
B   are diagnosed by urethroscopy.
C   rapidly cause upper renal tract damage.
D   are a recognized cause of oligohydramnios.
E   are diagnosed by micturating cysto-urethrogram.

11.21. A B C
Inappropriate ADH occurs in a number of unrelated conditions which include CNS infections and trauma, respiratory problems, drugs (vincristine) and malignant tumours (pancreas, Ewing's sarcoma). The serum sodium (and osmolality) is low whereas excretion of sodium in urine is continued. Urine output is diminished. Treatment consists of restriction of fluids and management of the primary condition. Hypertonic saline is usually of little benefit.

11.22. A C E
At birth less than 5% of normal boys have a fully retractable prepuce. By the age of 3 years the prepuce can be retracted in 90% of boys. The optimum age for circumcision is 6–12 months. Complications such as haemorrhage and infection are more likely to occur in the first week of life. Ammoniacal dermatitis is the commonest cause of meatal ulcer. Unless definite phimosis is present circumcision is not indicated at any age.

11.23. A B E
In penile hypospadias the chordee prevents the child from passing urine in the standing position as it would wet his legs. Though the urethra may be normal the meatus is often stenotic. Neonatal circumcision is contraindicated as the foreskin is often essential for repair later. There is no abnormality of the sphincters. Though sexual intercourse may be difficult, there is no impotence.

11.24. A C D E
Posterior urethral valves are sail-shaped membranes that arise from the verumontanum in males. Diagnosis is made by micturating cysto-urethrogram. Damage to the upper renal tract is caused by obstruction and vesicoureteric reflux which is often present. Oligohydramnios occurs because fetal urine is unable to get into the amniotic fluid.

11.25. Which of the following statements is/are true of undescended testes?

A   The average age at full descent is 1 year.
B   Retractile testes should be surgically fixed in the scrotum.
C   The testes are undescended at birth in more than 50% of male infants of less than 1500 g.
D   Ectopic testes should be excised.
E   An undescended testis should be brought down by operation by the age of 2 years.

11.26. Which of the following is/are more likely to occur in a patient with undescended testes?

A   Trauma to the testes.
B   Infertility.
C   Torsion of the testes.
D   Malignancy of the testes.
E   Testicular dysplasia.

11.27. Which of the following statements is/are correct?

A   A retractile testis may be found in the inguinal canal.
B   The cremasteric reflex is most active between the ages of 6 months and 4 years.
C   In unilateral cryptorchidism the undescended testis is usually larger than the descended one.
D   More than 50% of undescended testes diagnosed at birth, descend by the age of 1 year.
E   Malignancy is unlikely to occur in an undescended testis before the age of 5 years.

11.28. Which of the following statements is/are true?

A   In female pseudohermaphroditism the infant should be raised as a female irrespective of the appearance of the external genitalia.
B   In male pseudohermaphroditism the basis for decision for sex of rearing is largely determined by the morphology of the external genitalia.
C   The absolute guides for the sex of rearing are gonadal and chromosomal sex.
D   It is usually recommended that sex of rearing should not be altered after the age of 3 years irrespective of gonadal and chromosomal sex.
E   In the absence of ovary the fetal female genital system does not develop.

11.25. C E

The testis begins to descend at 28 weeks' gestation and is in the scrotum by 34 weeks' gestation (2 kg) in the majority of cases. The retractile testes retract into the inguinal canal in response to an exaggerated cremasteric reflex. They can be brought down by careful manipulation when the child is relaxed in a warm room. Ectopic testes are morphologically normal and therefore should not be excised. Most undescended testes that are likely to descend will do so by the end of the first year. Dysplastic changes are detectable in the testis by the end of the first year and continue to increase thereafter.

11.26. A B C D E

The undescended testis is dysplastic and atrophic which results in infertility. The risk of malignancy is 20–40% more than the normal testis. As the testis may be in the inguinal region there is an increased risk of trauma and torsion.

11.27. A B D E

The cremasteric reflex is weak or absent at birth and is most active between the ages of 6 months to 4 years. It is not abnormal for the testis to retract into the inguinal canal. Such testes adopt a permanent scrotal position at puberty. The undescended testis is usually atrophic and smaller than the descended one. The incidence of undescended testes in full-term infants at birth is 3.4% compared to 1% at 1 year. Though the incidence of malignancy in the adult population is increased by 40%, testicular malignancy in children under the age of 5 years is extremely rare.

11.28. A B D

As female pseudohermaphrodites have normal ovaries, fallopian tubes and uterus they are potentially fertile and therefore should be reared as females. Moreover the genital defect is readily corrected. It is desirable, if possible, to assign the sex of rearing in accordance with gonadal and chromosomal sex but these criteria are not absolute guides in making a decision especially in male pseudohermaphrodites when morphology of the external genitalia and the sensitivity of the phallus to androgens have to be taken into account. Whereas fetal testicular morphogenic hormones are essential for differentiation of male sex structures and for retrogression of the female ducts, a functioning fetal gonad is not a prerequisite for development of a female genital system.

12 Neurology and neurosurgery

12.1. Which of the following statements is/are true of cerebral palsy?
A   There has been a decrease in incidence in the last decade.
B   There is progressive neurological deterioration.
C   There is spontaneous improvement in motor function in some cases.
D   Mental retardation is present in more than 95% of cases.
E   They may have abnormal tonic neck patterns in the neonatal period.

12.2. A baby boy was born at 32 weeks' gestation. He smiled at 6 weeks and could pick up a small object with finger and thumb at 10 months. He is not yet walking at the age of 26 months. His speech is normal. Likely diagnoses is/are
A   mental subnormality.
B   cerebral palsy.
C   muscular dystrophy.
D   spina bifida occulta.
E   phenylketonuria.

12.3. A 3-year-old boy is found to be functioning at an 18-month level across all areas of development. History (including family history) and physical examination are unremarkable. Which of the following is/are true?
A   There is a greater than 75% chance that thorough investigation will reveal a cause.
B   The cerebral CT scan will be abnormal in more than 10% of such children.
C   The serum creatine kinase should be measured.
D   A chromosome study may show X-linked intellectual handicap to be the cause.
E   This child would not qualify for a handicapped child allowance until he reaches school age.

12.4. In complex partial seizures (psychomotor seizures, temporal lobe epilepsy) which of the following may occur as seizure manifestations?
A   Repeated swallowing.
B   Dream-like states.
C   Central abdominal pain.
D   Vertigo.
E   Oculogyric crises.

12.1. C E

The incidence of cerebral palsy has not decreased (in fact, might have increased because more premature infants with neurological problems are being saved) over the last decade. It is a static lesion though it may appear to be progressive because the symptoms may not manifest till later. Spontaneous improvement in motor function has been observed, particularly in premature infants. Intelligence may be normal but may present problems in assessment because of disturbance of motor function. Obligatory tonic neck patterns may be the only sign in the neonatal period.

12.2. B C

Other than gross motor ability the child is developing normally. He cannot have mental subnormality or phenylketonuria (which causes mental deficiency). Spina bifida occulta does not cause motor problems. Children with congenital dislocation of the hips will have an abnormal gait but there is no delay in walking. Cerebral palsy and muscular dystrophy are possible diagnoses.

12.3. C D

If diagnosis of mental deficiency cannot be established on history and physical examination, chances of it being diagnosed following investigations are small. The majority of patients with mental deficiency have a morphologically normal brain. 25% of children with Duchenne muscular dystrophy (diagnosed by measuring serum creatine kinase) have mental deficiency. In morphologically normal boys X-linked mental retardation is the commonest recognizable cause of mental deficiency.

12.4. A B C D

Complex partial seizures are due to epileptic discharges in the temporal lobes. Symptoms include confusion at the time of the attack without complete loss of consciousness, déjà vu dreamy states, visual and auditory hallucinations, mood disturbances (fear, anxiety, laughing, anger and aggression), semi-purposeful motor activities (motor automatisms, particularly repeated chewing and swallowing). Central abdominal pain (abdominal epilepsy) and vertigo are other manifestations. Oculogyric crisis do not occur.

12.5. Infantile spasms

A characteristically occur in the first year of life.
B are sometimes associated with a characteristic pattern on EEG.
C may occur in children with tuberous sclerosis.
D sometimes occur in previously normal children.
E are a benign seizure disorder.

12.6. Which of the following statements is/are true of simple febrile convulsions?

A The IQ of children with recurrent febrile convulsions is lower than their unaffected siblings.
B There is an increased risk of recurrence if the first fit occurs before the age of 1 year.
C An EEG is not indicated in the assessment for treatment of febrile convulsions.
D The risk of developing epilepsy later is 10 times that of the general population.
E Phenobarbitone should be administered regularly to all infants with febrile convulsions until the age of 3 years.

12.7. The frequency of recurrence of benign febrile convulsions in childhood can be reduced by

A the prophylactic administration of adequate doses of phenytoin sodium.
B the prophylactic administration of adequate doses of phenobarbital.
C the prophylactic administration of adequate doses of sodium valproate.
D the administration of carbamazepine during febrile illnesses.
E the administration of diazepam rectally regularly during febrile illnesses.

12.8 Some anticonvulsants may produce unwanted side effects when dosage and serum levels are within the recommended range. Which of the following examples illustrate this phenomenon?

A Phenytoin and diplopia.
B Phenobarbitone and severe drowsiness.
C Sodium valproate and liver toxicity.
D Carbamazepine and Stevens–Johnson syndrome.
E Phenobarbitone and hyperactivity.

12.5. A B C D
The age of onset of infantile spasms is 3–6 months but onset may occur as early as the neonatal period or as late as 2 years. They most commonly occur in association with neonatal asphyxia, birth trauma or previous meningitis. They are also seen in patients with tuberous sclerosis and may sometimes occur in previously normal children. Whooping cough vaccine has been implicated in its causation but the incidence is less than 1:150 000. Though they may remit spontaneously, other seizure types develop later in life in about 50% of patients and mental retardation has been reported in 80–90% of cases on long-term follow-up. The EEG changes when present are diagnostic (hypsarrhythmia).

12.6. B C
Febrile convulsions do not affect the IQ of children. The EEG is of little or no value in the assessment. The risk of developing epilepsy later is four times that of the general population. Phenobarbitone is administered regularly to infants who have three or more febrile convulsions but may have to be replaced with sodium valproate if side effects (hyperactivity) occur. The risk is increased if the first fit occurs before the age of 1 year.

12.7. B C E
Controlled trials have shown that prophylactic administration of phenobarbital, sodium valproate and administration of diazepam regularly during febrile illnesses reduces the frequency of occurrence of febrile convulsions. Phenytoin sodium and carbamazepine do not alter the frequency of febrile convulsions.

12.8 C D E
Central nervous system manifestations are the commonest with phenytoin (Dilantin) therapy and include cerebellar disturbances (nystagmus, ataxia and slurred speech), mental confusion and are the direct effect of the drug. Gingival hypertrophy will occur even when the drug is given in therapeutic dosages. Other toxic effects are skin rashes and bone marrow depression which are due to hypersensitivity. Initially phenobarbitone causes drowsiness which resolves spontaneously but hyperactivity may be troublesome even with therapeutic dosages. Sodium valproate causes liver toxicity which particulary occurs in the first 2–12 weeks after commencement of therapy. It is thought to be an idiosyncratic response. Carbamazepine therapy results in Stevens–Johnson syndrome in 3% of patients as a result of hypersensitivity.

12.9. Which of the following statements is/are true of benign febrile convulsions?

A   The diagnosis is not acceptable if the infant is less than 6 months.
B   The temperature is usually below 38°C.
C   There is increased incidence in patients with cerebral palsy.
D   The incidence is increased in siblings.
E   There are no focal signs following the seizure.

12.10. Childhood absence (petit mal) epilepsy

A   has a characteristic aura preceding an attack.
B   commonly responds to treatment with ethosuximide.
C   has characteristic 3 per second spike and wave discharge patterns on EEG.
D   characteristically commences between 4 and 10 years.
E   is caused by the pertussis component in triple antigen (DPT).

12.11. Which of the following statements is/are true of childhood absence epilepsy (petit mal)?

A   The presenting symptom may be poor school performance.
B   The diagnosis can be established on history even in the absence of EEG changes.
C   The peak incidence is 4–10 years.
D   The presence of grand mal seizures in the patient excludes such a diagnosis.
E   The drug of choice for treatment is phenytoin sodium.

12.12. An 18-month-old child on three occasions, each after minor trauma, has had episodes in which he has stiffened, become pale, given a cry, fallen on the ground, arched his back, rolled his eyes up and jerked, then has become limp, woken up and although a little groggy for a few minutes he then fully recovered. Which of the following is/are correct of this patient?

A   These attacks are not epileptic seizures.
B   These attacks require investigations with CT scan, and EEG and lumbar puncture.
C   This is a breath holding attack which the child is doing deliberately and ought to be punished.
D   These attacks are breath holding attacks and, to avoid brain damage, mouth-to-mouth resuscitation should be applied in any further attacks.
E   These attacks are syncopal (vasovagal, pale, breath holding) and though alarming they cause no damage.

12.9. A D E

By definition febrile convulsions occur in normal children over the age of 6 months and under the age of 5 years. The convulsions may occur at any temperature but usually it is above 38.5°C. There are no changes in the cerebrospinal fluid. There is increased familial incidence and there are no focal signs following the seizure.

12.10. B C D

The drug of choice for treatment of petit mal epilepsy is ethosuximide. It also responds to treatment with valproic acid and tridione. It commences between 4 and 10 years and is characterized by staring and arrest of activity. The EEG shows the characteristic 3 per second spike and wave pattern. There is rarely an aura preceding an attack and it has no relationship to pertussis vaccine.

12.11. A C

Repeated attacks of petit mal epilepsy will result in inattention and poor school performance. Without EEG changes the diagnosis cannot be established with certainty. Some children with petit mal epilepsy can also have concomitant grand mal seizures. The drug of choice for treatment is ethosuximide. The peak incidence is 4–10 years.

12.12. A E

The history suggests a child with vasovagal attacks which are not epileptic seizures. They do not require investigations or treatment. They are not deliberate and punishment will not resolve the problem.

12.13. Which of the following is/are true of meningitis in an 11-month-old infant?
A   It is most commonly caused by *Streptococcus pneumoniae*.
B   Neck stiffness may not be present.
C   It often presents with lethargy and refusal to feed.
D   Inappropriate antidiuretic hormone secretion is a recognized feature.
E   Subdural effusions are a recognized complication.

12.14. A 3-year-old boy presents with high fever, irritability and progressive loss of consciousness. Examination shows left VIth nerve palsy, bilateral papilloedema and right hemiparesis. Which of the following statements is/are true?
A   Immediate lumbar puncture is required.
B   The EEG would be abnormal.
C   Blood culture is indicated.
D   CAT scan is indicated.
E   Head ultrasound will establish the diagnosis.

12.15. Recognized causes of deafness include
A   meningitis.
B   chloroquine.
C   aminoglycosides.
D   neonatal hyperbilirubinaemia.
E   sulphadiazine.

12.16. Convergent squint
A   is less common than divergent squint in children.
B   is often associated with hypermetropia.
C   may be completely reversed by the use of spectacles.
D   often resolves spontaneously at the age of about 5 years.
E   is clinically significant principally because of its cosmetic effects.

12.13. B C D E

Physical signs of meningitis, viz. neck stiffness, Kernig's sign and bulging fontanelle may not be present in infants. The younger the infant the more likely it will present with lethargy and refusal to feed. The commonest organism in an 11-month-old infant is *Hameophilus influenzae*. Subdural effusions occur during the course of treatment and may require drainage in some cases. Inappropriate antidiuretic hormone secretion often occurs and is manifested by hyponatraemia. It is treated by restriction of fluids.

12.14. B C D

The history and physical examination suggest a diagnosis of a space-occupying lesion with raised intracranial pressure in the left hemisphere, possibly associated with infection. Lumbar puncture is dangerous as it may cause herniation of the medulla. The EEG would be abnormal and a CAT scan would accurately demonstrate the position and the nature of the lesion. Head ultrasound, though helpful, is not possible (fontanelle being closed) and therefore will not establish the diagnosis. Diagnosis is most likely a brain abscess and blood culture may isolate the organism.

12.15. A C D

Neonatal hyperbilirubinaemia and aminoglycosides cause sensorineural hearing loss. Complications of meningitis include cranial nerve involvement resulting in deafness, blindness, hemi- or quadriplegia, muscular hypotonia, ataxia and permanent seizure disorders. Chloroquine and sulphadiazine are not known to cause deafness.

12.16. B C

Convergent squint is more common than divergent squint and is often associated with hypermetropia which can be corrected by the use of suitable spectacles. Convergent squint if untreated can result in amblyopia. Treatment may have to be continued for a number of years and some children require surgery for a residual amount of crossing that cannot be controlled with glasses alone.

12.17. Which of the following statements about convergent squint is/are true?

A If surgery aligns the squinting eye, the vision in that eye usually improves spontaneously.

B Surgery should only be done after patching treatment has improved vision.

C Retinoblastoma and congenital glaucoma often present with convergent squint.

D When due to esotropia it is alternating.

E Convergent squint has a better visual prognosis than divergent squint.

12.18. A child of 18 months presents with a nonparalytic convergent squint. Which of the following statements is/are true?

A The squinting eye moves to fix vision when the normal eye is covered.

B Hypermetropia is the most likely cause.

C Hypermetropia if present will improve with age.

D The squint will improve with age.

E The squinting eye should be occluded as part of the orthoptic treatment.

12.19. Which of the following statements about amblyopia is/are true?

A It is treatable until the age of 20 years.

B It is treatable until the age of 4 years.

C It is treated by alternately occluding the good and the bad eye.

D It is usually caused by squint or anisometropia.

E It is a cause of an afferent pupillary defect.

12.20. Which of the following is/are recognized causes of cataracts in child-hood?

A Galactosaemia.

B Gaucher's disease.

C Congenital rubella.

D Down's syndrome.

E Cystic fibrosis.

12.17. B C

Most cases of convergent squint are due to disturbances of vision such as hypermetropia which requires treatment with glasses or topical myotics. Aligning the squinting eye by surgery will not restore vision. The majority of patients will respond to treatment with glasses though some may require surgery for a residual amount of squint. Retinoblastoma and congenital glaucoma cause visual disturbance which leads to convergent squint. A divergent squint has better prognosis than convergent squint. When due to esotropia it is alternating and refractive errors are uncommon.

12.18. A C D E

Convergent squint is usually due to refractive errors but at age 18 months does not produce diplopia. When the normal eye is covered, the squinting eye moves in order to allow the patient to look at the object clearly. Other causes include visual defects such as cataracts and refractive errors. Though hypermetropia requires treatment with glasses, it improves with age. Only the normal eye is occluded for treatment.

12.19. B D

Susceptibility to amblyopia is greatest within the first 3 years of life and the risk lasts till full visual potential and stability have been achieved. Hence treatment of cases after the age of 4 years is unsatisfactory. Treatment consists of occluding the good eye. Anisometropia results in squint in order to suppress the image of the deviating eye and to avoid diplopia. If it is untreated it would result in amblyopia. There is no disturbance of pupillary reflex in amblyopia.

12.20. A C D

In galactosaemia there are raised levels of galacticol which causes cataracts. In congenital rubella, infection of the lens causes the development of cataracts. Children with Down's syndrome are more likely to develop cataracts. There is no increase of cataracts in infants with Gaucher's disease or cystic fibrosis.

12.21. Which of the following is/are true in relation to mental retardation?
A   Mental retardation occurs in more than 1% of the population.
B   The majority of mildly retarded individuals are at the upper end of socioeconomic scale.
C   Dietary modification may prevent some forms of mental retardation.
D   Pregnant women with no immunity against rubella should be immunized as soon as they find out they are pregnant.
E   Early treatment of congenital hypothryoidism may not prevent the associated mental retardation.

12.22. Which of the following statements is/are correct of neuromuscular diseases?
A   The Duchenne and Becker types of muscular dystrophy exhibit the same mode of inheritance.
B   Visible fasciculations are characteristic of the muscular dystrophies.
C   Distal distribution of weakness and sensory loss is characteristic of peripheral neuropathies.
D   Nerve conduction velocity studies are useful in the diagnosis of spinal muscular atrophy.
E   The serum creatine kinase level is always elevated in the early stages of Duchenne type muscular dystrophy.

12.23. A distended fontanelle is a characteristic feature in infants suffering from
A   communicating hydrocephalus.
B   meningitis.
C   non-communicating hydrocephalus.
D   vitamin A intoxication.
E   megalencephaly.

12.24. An 18-month-old baby presents with a 10-day history of refusal to walk and ill-defined pain in the legs. On examination he cries when his legs are moved and will not flex his lumbar spine. Tendon reflexes are brisk. ESR = 30 mm/1 hr. Total white cell count = 20 000/cmm (65% neutrophils, 25% lymphocytes, 8% monocytes, 2% eosinophils). Which of the following diagnosis/es is/are likely?
A   Neuroblastoma.
B   Infective polyneuritis.
C   Poliomyelitis.
D   Lumbar discitis.
E   Osteomyelitis of spine.

12.21. A C E

Mental retardation can be defined as a performance more than 2 standard deviations below the mean. It follows that 3% of the population will fall in this category. The majority of mildly retarded individuals are at the lower end of the socioeconomic scale which suggests influence of environment. Mental retardation can be prevented by diet in many metabolic diseases: examples are phenylketonuria and galactosaemia. Rubella immunization should not be carried out in pregnant women as rubella embryopathy though rare has been observed following immunization during pregnancy. Though early treatment of congenital hypothyroidism will result in normal development in most patients, it does not prevent mental retardation in all cases.

12.22. A C E

The Duchenne and Becker types of muscular dystrophy are both sex-linked recessive. Fasciculations are characteristic of motor neurone disease. In peripheral neuropathies there is weakness and sensory loss distally. In spinal muscular atrophy, electromyography shows evidence of denervation of muscle including low potentials and fasciculations. Nerve conduction studies are within normal range. In Duchenne muscular dystrophy the serum creatine kinase level is raised at birth and is ten times the normal value at the age of 1 month.

12.23. A B C D

A distended fontanelle is seen in infants with communicating hydrocephalus, meningitis, non-communicating hydrocephalus and vitamin A intoxication (due to raised intracranial pressure). The fontanelle is normal in megalencephaly.

12.24. A D E

Pain in the legs and lumbar spine in neuroblastoma occurs due to bony metastasis. In infected polyneuritis and poliomyelitis there is pain on pressure on the muscles but no pain in the spine. Lumbar discitis and osteomyelitis of the spine can result in local pain due to the inflammation and referred pain in the legs due to nerve root compression.

12.25. Abnormal EEGs are usually seen in
A   childhood absence epilepsy (petit mal).
B   infantile spasms.
C   in between breath-holding attacks.
D   Jacksonian epilepsy.
E   behaviour disorders.

12.26. Migraine consists of attacks of headache, characteristically associated with which of the following?
A   Visual field defect.
B   Neck rigidity.
C   Intolerance of noise.
D   Unilateral Horner's syndrome.
E   Vomiting.

12.27. Which of the following statements is/are true of cerebral oedema due to head injury?
A   Fluid intake should be restricted.
B   It is aggravated by retention of carbon dioxide.
C   It is aggravated by administration of corticosteroids.
D   It is associated with a fall in blood pressure.
E   It is associated with bradycardia.

12.28. Parents who have had one baby with meningomyelocele seek advice about risks to future offspring. Which of the following statements is/are true?
A   Amniocentesis for alpha fetoprotein in the next pregnancy at 15 weeks will be diagnostically informative.
B   Chorionic villus sampling at 9 weeks' gestation will be diagnostically informative.
C   Any increase in risk relates only to meningomyelocele.
D   The risk for neural tube defect is approximately 5%.
E   A history that one of mother's siblings had anencephaly would alter the risk.

12.25. A B D
EEG changes are characteristic in petit mal epilepsy (3 per second spike and wave), infantile spasms (hypsarrhythmia) and Jacksonian epilepsy. EEG is normal in patients with breath-holding attacks in between attacks (though there is slowing during the attack) and has no characteristic features in behaviour disorders.

12.26. A C E
Classically, an attack of migraine is preceded by an aura which often consists of transient visual disturbances including field defects and zig-zag lines. Other symptoms include intolerance of noise, photophobia and vomiting. Neck rigidity and unilateral Horner's syndrome are not features of migraine.

12.27. A B D E
Cerebral oedema due to head injury should be treated by restriction of fluids to two-third of maintenance requirements. Carbon dioxide retention causes vasodilatation and thereby aggravates the cerebral oedema. Corticosteroids may help to reduce cerebral oedema. Fall in blood pressure and bradycardia are recognized signs of raised intracranial pressure.

12.28. A D E
Amniotic fluid alpha fetoprotein measurements are reliable in predicting open neural tube defects. Chorionic villus biopsy will not help to make an in utero diagnosis of meningomyelocele. Siblings of meningomyelocele infants are at risk of having anencephaly. The inheritance of neural tube defects is polygenic (multifactorial) and therefore the risk is approximately 5%. The risks are increased if the mother's siblings have had anencephaly.

12.29. With regard to spina bifida (myelocele)

A   prenatal diagnosis is possible.
B   the majority of cases develop hydrocephalus.
C   severe kyphosis and scoliosis are adverse predictive features.
D   reflex activity is characteristically absent below the neurological level of the lesion.
E   the autonomic nervous system is not involved.

12.30. Which of the following situations is/are common reasons for operative intervention in the management of children with spina bifida?

A   Development of genitourinary complications.
B   Development of hydrocephalus.
C   Orthopaedic deformity of the lower limbs.
D   Restriction of movement of the thoracic cage.
E   Onset of acute bowel obstruction.

12.31. In a patient with hydrocephalus controlled by a shunt, which of the following may be produced by blockage of the shunt?

A   Papilloedema.
B   Headache.
C   Fits.
D   Irritability.
E   Failure to progress at school.

12.32. In the presence of raised intracranial pressure there may be

A   bradycardia.
B   bilateral sixth nerve palsy.
C   arterial hypertension.
D   no history of headache.
E   no papilloedema in a newborn infant.

12.29. A B C
In spina bifida prenatal diagnosis is possible by ultrasound or by measuring alpha fetoprotein. The majority of cases develop hydrocephalus because of Arnold–Chiari malformation. Abnormalities of the spine indicate that the lesion is high and therefore the prognosis is poor. Reflex activity is present below the neurological level of the lesion and the autonomic nervous system is involved.

12.30. A B C
Operative treatment is necessary for patients with spina bifida with genito-urinary complications to prevent recurrent urinary tract infection, for hydro-cephalus to prevent raised intracranial pressure and correction of ortho-paedic deformities in order to make the patient mobile. There is no treat-ment recommended for restriction of thoracic cage movements and acute bowel obstruction will respond to enemas and washouts.

12.31. A B C D E
A blocked shunt would lead to raised intracranial pressure and could present with papilloedema, headache, fits, irritability and failure to progress at school.

12.32. A B C D E
Bradycardia and arterial hypertension are recognized signs of raised intracra-nial pressure. Sixth nerve palsy is due to the stretching of the nerve because of its long intracranial course. Patients with raised intracranial pressure may not have any headache. In the newborn infant there is no papilloedema because the sutures will separate thereby accommodating the raised intracra-nial pressure.

13   Psychiatry and social medicine

13.1. Common causes of school refusal in a 5-year-old include
A   phobia about the school.
B   schizophrenia.
C   parental marital problems.
D   depression in the mother.
E   depression in the child.

13.2. School refusal in an adolescent may result from
A   separation anxiety.
B   schizophrenia.
C   anorexia nervosa.
D   severe depression.
E   delinquency.

13.3. Symptoms associated with anxiety in childhood include
A   excessive worrying and fears in normal social situations.
B   early morning wakening.
C   pseudo-maturity.
D   poor sense of self-esteem.
E   attention-seeking behaviour.

13.4. Elective surgical operations should be avoided in children aged 1–3 years because
A   the infant is immunologically vulnerable at that time.
B   some congenital malformations may not have been detected.
C   they may induce infantile autism.
D   the danger of separation trauma is highest at that time.
E   anaesthetic risks are higher.

13.1. C D

Causes of school refusal include parental marital problems and depression in the mother. Young children are rarely fearful of the school itself. Unlike adolescents, in a 5-year-old child depression and schizophrenia do not present as school refusal.

13.2. A B D

School refusal is a condition in which a fear of going to school is the superficial aspect of a fear of leaving the parent. In adolescents it is also associated with depression and may be a presenting symptom of schizophrenia. Delinquency can result in truancy but not school phobia. School refusal is not a feature of anorexia nervosa.

13.3. A C D E

A small amount of worry is normal in any new social situation but excessive worrying and fears are manifestation of anxiety. The child is often shy, timid and clinging, emotionally immature, overdependent and has attention-seeking behaviour and poor self-esteem. He often pretends to be more confident and competent than he really feels. Sleep problems are rare.

13.4. D

Above the age of 1 year the younger the child the more severe the distress of hospitalization is until the age of 3 years when it diminishes. Immunity of infants is lowest at the age of 3–6 months. There is no relationship between infantile autism and hospitalization. Anaesthetic risks are no greater at this age than at other ages. It is irrelevant whether other congenital malformations may not have been detected.

13.5. Clinical depression in childhood

A is often masked by psychosomatic or conduct symptoms.

B is associated with withdrawal, isolation and loss of interest in usual activities.

C is rarely associated with sleep disorder.

D may lead to thoughts about death or suicide.

E may be associated with hallucinations and delusions.

13.6. Which of the following statements is/are true of tricyclic antidepressants?

A They are one of the major causes of fatal accidental poisoning in children.

B They usually provide only temporary relief of nocturnal enuresis.

C They are the treatment of choice for reactive depression.

D They are more cardiotoxic in children than in adults.

E They exert a 'paradoxical effect' on hyperactivity.

13.7. Which of the following statements is/are true of breath-holding attacks?

A Consciousness is not lost.

B Clonic twitching may occur.

C Anticonvulsant treatment is indicated when frequency of attacks exceeds once a week.

D Onset is rarely before the age of 12 months.

E Ventricular asystole is an inconstant but recognized feature.

13.8. Which of the following statements is/are applicable in a 6-year-old who has temper tantrums?

A Should be smacked.

B Should be allowed to have his way.

C Should have 'time out' for at least an hour.

D Should be ignored.

E Should have 'time out' for the duration of the tantrum.

13.5. B D E
Depression results in a sense of lack of pleasure in life which results in withdrawal, isolation and loss of interest in usual activities, and persistent lowering of mood which leads to thoughts about death or suicide. In severe cases of endogenous depresson it is associated with hallucinations and delusions. Sleep disorders (insomnia or hypersomnia) are common. There are no psychosomatic or conduct symptoms.

13.6. A B
Tricyclic antidepressants cause cardiac arrhythmias, have no antidote and can result in fatal accidental poisoning in children. Therapy in nocturnal enuresis results in temporary improvement and the problem may recur even while the child is on treatment and very often following cessation of treatment. They are almost as effective as stimulants in hyperactivity. Cardiotoxicity is the same in adults and children. For treatment of reactive depression they should be reserved for those who do not respond to psychotherapy.

13.7. B E
In breath-holding attacks, convulsions and loss of consciousness can result and signal the end of an attack. Ventricular asystole, though rare, may occur. Anticonvulsants do not prevent the attacks. Onset can occur at any age.

13.8. D E
Tantrums are a manifestation of attention-seeking behaviour and they are best managed by ignoring or by 'time out' for the duration of the temper. Punishment (smacking) or reward (allowing the child to have its own way) will perpetuate the problem as the child has been able to get 'attention'. The period of 'time out' is not fixed but is dependent on the duration of the tantrum and the age of the child.

13.9. Truancy is often accompanied by
A antisocial behaviour.
B separation anxiety.
C recurrent abdominal pain.
D poor peer relationships.
E panic attacks.

13.10. Stealing by 5-year-old children
A is sometimes learned from parents.
B usually leads to delinquency.
C commonly occurs at home.
D is uncommon.
E is a sign of parental neglect.

13.11. Behaviour therapy in children may utilize which of the following principles?
A Reinforcement
B Transference.
C Free association.
D Time out.
E Resistance.

13.12. The principle features of hyperactivity include
A poor concentration.
B hypersomnia.
C obesity.
D impulsiveness.
E restlessness.

13.9. A D

Truancy is a form of antisocial behaviour in older children and adolescents. It is often accompanied by other antisocial activities such as drug taking and sexual offences (including sexual abuse of younger children) and poor peer relationships. It is not a manifestation of emotional disorders which include separation anxiety, recurrent abdominal pain and panic attacks. However, an emotional disorder may coexist.

13.10. A C E

Stealing sometimes occurs in children of parents who boast of breaking the law (e.g. avoiding tax or exceeding speed limits). It commonly occurs at home, sometimes to invite punishment or attention as the child has a feeling of not being cared for. It occurs equally in all social groups. Almost all children steal something at some time during childhood.

13.11. A D

Principles of behaviour therapy include extinction (withdrawal of love or attention, material goods), punishment (to choose to remove undesirable behaviour), reinforcement (rewarding a good behaviour), and ignoring ('time-out'). Free association, transference and resistance are technical terms relating to psychodynamic forms of psychotherapy.

13.12. A D E

In infants the clinical features of hyperactivity include difficulty in feeding and sleeping poorly and irregularly. In children it is manifested as restlessness, inability to concentrate (e.g. doing puzzles, construction toys) and impulsiveness. They may also be irritable and moody. Obesity is not a feature of hyperactivity.

13.13. Good prognostic signs in a child with a conduct disorder include
A   poor self-esteem.
B   poor social skills.
C   good scholastic aptitude.
D   success at sports.
E   development of a stable relationship or friendship.

13.14. Possible causative mechanisms for conduct disorders in childhood include
A   psychosocial adversity.
B   inadequate socialization.
C   pregnancy and birth complications.
D   inherited difficult temperament.
E   multiple separations from parents.

13.15. Which of the following statements is/are true of early onset of psychosis (infantile autism)?
A   Onset occurs before the age of 30 months.
B   It is a disorder of communication.
C   Signs include lack of eye contact.
D   A well-developed delusional system is apparent.
E   There is avoidance of human relationships.

13.16. A 4-year-old non-speaking child is referred because of overall cognitive retardation. He makes no eye contact, does not respond to his name and panics at the sound of a lawn-mower outside. He is hyperactive and walks on tip-toe, spinning a piece of string between his fingers. Which of the following is/are correct?
A   The patient will be disturbed if his familiar routines are interrupted.
B   The condition has been precipitated by acute intracranial infection.
C   Prognosis with psychotherapy is good.
D   The condition is more common in boys.
E   There is a strong familial tendency.

13.13. C D E

Children whose antisocial behaviour is limited to minor delinquency or isolated delinquency acts, whose relationships with other children are good, who are good at sports and show good scholastic aptitude have a better prognosis as each of these can be the basis of self-esteem and social skills development. Poor social skills and self-esteem are indicators of bad prognosis.

13.14. A B C D E

Epidemiological studies have shown that all the factors mentioned increase the incidence of conduct disorders.

13.15. A B C E

Infantile autism usually presents before the age of 30 months. Such infants have abnormal development of social relationships and language (leading to disorder of communication, lack of eye contact and avoidance of human relationships). Delusions are not a feature of infantile autism.

13.16. A D

The stem suggests a diagnosis of infantile autism which is more common in boys. Such patients get distressed and agitated if their familiar routines are interrupted. It has no relationship to intracranial infection. Though the condition can be familial (2–3% of sibs are affected), the aetiology is heterogenous. The prognosis with or without treatment is poor.

13.17. Which of the following is/are recognized features of anorexia nervosa in adolescent girls?
A   Amenorrhoea.
B   Hyperthyroidism.
C   Physical hyperactivity.
D   Fluid and electrolyte abnormalities.
E   A normal perception of body size.

13.18. Anorexia nervosa
A   only responds to family and individual psychotherapy.
B   is more common in girls than boys.
C   is influenced by community values about diet and thinness.
D   is easily confused with endogenous depression.
E   occurs less frequently in socially disadvantaged groups.

13.19. The differential diagnosis of a 14-year-old girl presenting with severe weight loss and amenorrhoea includes
A   depression.
B   anorexia nervosa.
C   anxiety.
D   bulimia.
E   subacute sclerosing panencephalitis (SSPE).

13.20. Child physical abuse and/or neglect should be suspected if
A   there is a delay in social and language skills with normal motor development.
B   there is growth failure without an organic cause.
C   a child is demanding and aggressive in the presence of his/her parents.
D   parents' history of injury in a child is not compatible with findings on examination.
E   the child continues to fail to thrive in hospital.

13.17. A C D
Clinical features of anorexia nervosa include excessive dieting because of a morbid fear of being fat and accompanying this there is frequently a misperception of bodily appearance (patient overestimating the size of thighs etc. in comparison with other children) and amenorrhoea. Electrolyte imbalance results from vomiting from water overloading and from abuse of diuretics or laxatives. Thyroid function is normal, though there is physical hyperactivity, e.g. fidgety and tremulous.

13.18. B C
Anorexia nervosa is more than 10 times as common in girls than in boys and is more common in communities where there is great emphasis on body image. Treatment consists of individual and family psychotherapy, behaviour modification techniques and nutritional rehabilitation. Hospitalization may be indicated. Depression is not a primary feature of anorexia nervosa. The condition can affect all social groups equally.

13.19. A B
In depression and anorexia nervosa there is severe weight loss and amenorrhoea. Amenorrhoea is not a feature of anxiety and subacute sclerosing panencephalitis. In bulimia there may be great fluctuations in weight (of more than 10–20 kg).

13.20. A B D
Children who are neglected tend to have delay in language and social skills because of lack of stimulation, they gain weight inadequately but put on weight when they are admitted and observed in hospital. Normal children can be demanding and aggressive. Classically in child abuse the history given by the parents is incompatible with the child's injuries.

13.21. The parents of a girl who has been sexually abused should be advised

A   that the child should talk about the incident until they have got it out of their system.
B   that what happened was not her fault.
C   to make sure that further incidents do not occur.
D   that they will have to reassure their daughter of her worth and their love.
E   that the girl will have to give testimony in open court if the perpetrator is charged.

13.22. The persistence for years of incest between father and daughter is frequently due to which of the following?

A   Coercion by the mother.
B   The child's fear she will not be believed.
C   The child's wish to protect her father from punishment.
D   The child's fear that revelation will lead to the break-up of the family.
E   The child's trust in her father.

13.23. Children who have been sexually abused frequently experience problems with

A   ability to trust others.
B   guilt.
C   poor self-esteem.
D   soiling.
E   problem of gender identity.

13.24. Enuresis in an 8-year-old boy who has been continent of urine between the ages of 4 and 5 years

A   may be precipitated by family crisis.
B   does not require specific treatment.
C   may have an organic cause.
D   may lead to poor self-esteem.
E   responds best to individual psychotherapy.

13.21. B C D

In child sexual abuse it is important that the child be reassured that it was not her fault, and the parents still love her and hold her in high esteem. It is important to make sure that further incidents do not occur. If the child is asked to testify it is usually held in a closed court. Repeated talking of the incident will make the child feel guilty and embarrassed.

13.22. B C D

In the majority of cases, the mother is unaware of the incest. Children are extremely loyal to their family and are afraid that they may cause break-down of the family if they mention it to other people. Often children's early attempts to draw attention to the problem are half-hearted and because they are met with anger and denial they do not persist. Most children lose all trust in the parent that is abusing them.

13.23. A B C

Sexually abused children have difficulty in trusting others as they have lost trust in a close family member, they feel guilty as they feel they are perpetuating the relationship and have poor self-esteem because of the fact that they feel valueless other than as a sex object. Soiling can occur but is not frequent. There is no problem with gender identity.

13.24. A C D

Enuresis in a child who has been continent before requires investigations. It can be precipitated by family crisis or may be the manifestation of some other disease such as urinary tract infection or diabetes mellitus. In the latter case the polyuria results in nocturnal enuresis though the child can cope with it during the day. Psychotherapy will be of very little use in such cases. These children have poor self-esteem. Treatment will depend on the cause.

13.25. Which of the following is/are correct?

A   Nocturnal enuresis is more frequent in boys than girls.
B   Diurnal enuresis is more frequent in boys than girls.
C   Nocturnal enuresis is more frequent in first-born children.
D   Nocturnal enuresis is a familial disorder.
E   Primary enuresis may present at the age of approximately 4 years.

13.26. In idiopathic megacolon (reservoir syndrome)

A   onset occurs usually from birth.
B   growth is delayed.
C   soiling occurs in more than 60% of cases.
D   there is a failure to pass formed bowel movements except by enema.
E   the rectum is often filled with faeces.

13.27. Completed suicide in childhood and adolescence

A   is more common in girls.
B   rarely occurs before the age of 10 years.
C   is usually accidental rather than being planned.
D   may be associated with drug or alcohol abuse.
E   is more likely if there is a family history of suicide or depression.

13.28. Obsessive-compulsive disorder in childhood

A   is fundamentally different to obsessive-compulsive disorder in adult-hood.
B   responds well to psychotherapy.
C   responds partially to behaviour therapy.
D   interferes with the development of social relationships.
E   is more common in families where the parents are also obsessional.

13.25. A C D
Epidemiological studies have shown nocturnal enuresis is more common in boys and in first-born children. It has a familial incidence. By definition primary enuresis is present from birth. Diurnal enuresis is more common in girls.

13.26. C E
In idiopathic megacolon there is voluntary retention of stool. Soiling occurs as a result of overflow incontinence. The child may pass small amounts of stool. Rectal examination shows hard stools in the rectum. There is no disturbance of growth. Though commonly seen in preschool children, it may present in infancy but is not present from birth.

13.27. B D E
Suicide in children under the age of 12 years is very rare. It is 3 times more common in adolescent boys than girls. Parents often suffer from psychiatric problems, especially depressive syndrome and personality disorders. It is usually planned and may be associated with drug or alcohol abuse.

13.28. A C D E
Obsessive-compulsive disorders in childhood are no different from those in adults. They respond best to tricyclic antidepressants, partially to behaviour therapy and not to psychotherapy. There is a strong family history with two-thirds of parents showing obsessional tendency and about 5% obsessional disorders. Twin studies suggest a genetic influence in obsessive personality traits. Rituals may seriously interfere with socialization and to development of peer and family relationships.

13.29. The first child of a young woman has been born with signs of Down's syndrome. When her medical attendant tells her and her husband the diagnosis, she rejects it angrily. Which of the following comments is/are appropriate?

A   This kind of reaction is abnormal.
B   This reaction is a manifestation of the defence mechanism of denial.
C   The mother should be left alone until she is able to accept the truth.
D   A series of interviews are necessary to help the mother to accept the diagnosis.
E   There is a genetic association between maternal psychopathology and Down's syndrome.

13.30. A 6-year-old boy with normal hearing and no physical abnormalities speaks appropriately at home but says nothing at school either in the classroom or in the playground. Which of the following is/are correct?

A   It is likely that he has been disturbed by psychological trauma at school.
B   The condition is due to reactive depression.
C   Speech therapy is of limited value in this condition.
D   The child's mutism is elective.
E   This speech disorder is indicative of early infantile autism.

13.31. Adolescents with chronic physical illness

A   experience more psychotic episodes than healthy adolescents.
B   more often experience loss of personal control and independence than do healthy adolescents.
C   are less likely to comply with treatment than are chronically ill children.
D   cope better with their limitations if their family life is stable.
E   have poor self-esteem in more than 80% of cases.

13.32. Which of the following statements is/are true of night terrors?

A   They usually indicate severe emotional disturbance.
B   They are accompanied by frightening dreams.
C   The child cannot remember much about them the next morning.
D   They occur in non-REM sleep.
E   They persist into early childhood.

13.29. B D

The normal reaction to bad news is first one of denial followed by bitterness and anger which is a defence mechanism of denial. The mother will need repeated interviews to help her to cope with the problem. There is no association between maternal psychopathology and Down's syndrome.

13.30. C D

The stem suggests a diagnosis of elective mutism. The condition is not usually caused by problems at school, reactive depression or early infantile autism. It does not require speech therapy. These children are often somewhat anxious and have an overprotective family.

13.31. B C E

Adolescents with chronic illness are more likely than children to be intolerant of the enforced dependency, particularly if their families do not appreciate how the illness interrupts their progress towards independence. Not complying with treatment is one way they may try to assert themselves as they feel loss of independence which results in loss of self-esteem. There is no increase in psychotic episodes.

13.32. C D

Night terrors and sleep walking occur in about 3% of children. The peak age is 4–7 years and the condition is self-limiting. The episodes occur in a period of arousal from EEG stages 3 and 4 sleep (non-REM sleep) so that the child is quite deeply asleep when showing the behaviour. There is a strong family history and the condition may be inherited as an autosomal dominant. They are more likely to occur if the child has had a stressful event the previous day but if they occur without symptoms they are not in themselves an indication of emotional disturbance. There are usually no accompanying frightening dreams.

14 Orthopaedics and musculoskeletal system

14.1. The upper age limit at which spontaneous resolution occurs is
A   3 years for bow legs.
B   4 years for outset hips.
C   5 years for internal tibial torsion.
D   9 years for knock knees.
E   more than 7 years for inset hips.

14.2. Which of the following statements is/are true in infants and children?
A   Newborn infants have flat feet.
B   Bow legs are normal in infants.
C   Knock knees are normal at 3–4 years of age.
D   Hallux valgus may be symptomatic.
E   Curly toes are familial.

14.3. Bilateral knock knee or genu valgum is
A   a normal limb posture from 2–6 years.
B   often unilateral.
C   painless.
D   best monitored by serial X-rays.
E   usually treated by splinting.

14.4. Talipes calcaneovalgus is of clinical significance because of its frequent association with
A   congenital heart disease.
B   syndactyly.
C   cleft palate.
D   congenital dislocation of the hip.
E   urogenital malformation.

14.1. A E
Infants are born with bow legs which straighten by the age of 2 years leading on to knock knees which resolve by the age of 6 years. Medial tibial torsion will not correct spontaneously after the age of 7 years. Inset hips continue to mould till the age of 16 years. Outset hips require orthopaedic treatment after the age of 3 years.

14.2. A B C D E
Newborn infants do not have well-developed foot arches and the feet appear flat. At birth the infant has bow legs. By the age of 12–24 months the legs have straightened and progress to knock knee. Adult configuration of legs is achieved by the age of 6–7 years. Hallux valgus is seen in adolescents especially in girls and is usually symptomless. The condition is progressive and may represent faulty development of the bones. Curly toes (some toes on top of others) are familial and are of no clinical significance.

14.3. A C
Infants have bow legs at birth which straighten by the age of 24 months and progress to knock knees. Persistence of knock knees beyond 6 years is abnormal and needs evaluation for an underlying abnormality. They do not require any investigations or treatment. The condition is bilateral. It is painless and requires no X-rays.

14.4. D
Talipes calcaneovalgus usually occurs because of the position of the fetus in utero which is also associated with congenital dislocation of the hip. There is no association between congenital heart disease, syndactyly, cleft palate and urogenital malformations with talipes calcaneovalgus.

14.5. Which of the following signs may be present in an infant with normal hips?
A   Asymmetrical thigh folds.
B   One leg kicks more freely.
C   One leg held in a position of external rotation and flexion.
D   Crying on movement of one leg.
E   Absent femoral pulses.

14.6. Which of the following are associated with increase in risk of congenital dislocation of hip?
A   Family history of the lesion.
B   Breech delivery.
C   Talipes calcaneovalgus.
D   Carrying the baby on the back in a sling with hips abducted.
E   Myelomeningocele.

14.7. Which of the following statements is/are true about slipped femoral epiphysis?
A   Peak incidence is between 5 and 10 years of age.
B   Bilaeral slipping occurs in 15–30% of cases.
C   Operative fixation of the epiphysis is the treatment of choice in early epiphyseal displacement to prevent further slipping.
D   Two-thirds of patients are known to have had clicks on abduction of the hips in the neonatal period.
E   Avascular necrosis is a recognized complication.

14.8. Perthes' disease is
A   often manifest by knee pain.
B   most commonly seen after puberty.
C   a form of avascular necrosis.
D   is indistinguishable from transient synovitis at the onset.
E   usually treated by surgery.

14.5. A B C D E
Ortolani manoevre is used to diagnose dislocation of the hips. Asymmetrical thigh folds should alert the examiner about the possibility of a dislocated hip though they may be present normally. The dislocated hips are held in abduction and extension. They do not cause pain. Absent femoral pulses may be found in coarctation of the aorta in an infant with normal hips. Foot and knee movements are normal.

14.6. A B C E
Aetiology of congenital dislocation of the hip is multifactorial. There are genetic factors and girls are more commonly affected than boys. It may be associated with other abnormalities such as talipes calcaneovalgus and myelomeningocele. Its association with breech is related to the position of the fetus in utero. The incidence has been shown to be less common in populations that carry their infants on the back in a sling with hips abducted, but is more common when carrying on a papoose board.

14.7. B C E
Slipped femoral epiphysis occurs in adolescent obese boys and is often bilateral. Avascular necrosis may occur as a result of disturbance of blood supply. There is no relationship to clicks on abduction of the hips in the neonatal period. Early fixation of the epiphysis will prevent further slipping.

14.8. A C D
Perthes' disease is an avascular necrosis of the femoral head at the age of 5–10 years. It presents with limp and pain at the hip joint or referred pain at the knee joint and may be indistinguishable from transient synovitis at the outset because the symptoms and X-ray changes are similar. Treatment consists of allowing the child to weight-bear but with the femur in an abducted position so that the head is well contained in the acetabulum. This is usually achieved by long-leg cast with the legs held in abduction and medial rotation by a bar between the two casts (Petrie cast) though surgical procedures have been developed to keep the femoral head contained in relation to the acetabulum.

14.9. Which of the following may cause a limp and a painful knee in a child?
A Perthes' disease.
B Slipped femoral epiphysis.
C Poliomyelitis.
D Haemophilia.
E Tuberculosis of hip joint.

14.10. Idiopathic scoliosis
A does not usually progress after skeletal maturity.
B is more common in girls than boys.
C has a familial tendency.
D usually presents with pain.
E is usually accompanied by rotation around the vertebra.

14.11. Which of the following statements is/are true of idiopathic scoliosis?
A The lateral curve of spine is accompanied by rotation around the vertebrae.
B It is accompanied by low back pains.
C Curve progression slows or stops with skeletal maturation.
D Bracing is best instituted at the time of skeletal maturity.
E Serial X-rays (at 4–6 month intervals) are required to observe the progression of scoliosis.

14.12. Which of the following statements is/are true of torticollis due to sternomastoid contracture?
A Restriction of rotation occurs towards the contracted side.
B Jaw tilt occurs away from the contracted side.
C Flattening of the face on the non-contracted side is observed.
D It is not seen in babies delivered by Caesarian section.
E Spinal abnormalities are found in more than 30% of cases.

14.9. A B D E
Disease in the hip joint can cause referred pain at the knee. Therefore Perthes' disease, slipped femoral epiphysis, tuberculosis of the hip joint and bleeding into the joint in haemophilia can all present with limp and pain in the knee. In poliomyelitis there is no involvement of the hip joint.

14.10. A B C E
The aetiology of idiopathic scoliosis is multifactorial. Some cases are autosomal dominant with incomplete penetrance. It is asymptomatic, is familial and is more common in girls. It continues to progress until growth ceases. The lateral curve of the spine is accompanied by a rotation around the vertebrae and the ribs rotate posteriourly on the convexity.

14.11. A C
There are two main elements to a scoliotic curve. Lateral deviation is a result of wedging of the vertebral bodies and discs. Rotation of vertebral bodies occurs around a vertical axis towards the convexity and the spinal processes towards the concavity of the curve. The progression of scoliosis stops or slows when growth ceases (only severe cases will progress) and therefore bracing would be of very little use at this stage. It is asymptomatic. As progress can be followed by periodic physical examination, serial X-rays are not necessary.

14.12. A B
In congenital torticollis the head is tilted towards the side of the contracture and the chin is turned towards the opposite side. There is restriction of rotation of neck towards the contracted side. Persistent torticollis may lead to asymmetrical development of the face and skull and results in poor development on the contracted side. Spinal abnormalities may cause torticollis but are not necessarily associated with congenital torticollis due to sternomastoid contracture. Torticollis has been observed in infants delivered by Caesarian section.

14.13. Which of the following statements is/are true of a sternomastoid tumour in a 6-week-old infant?

A   It will resolve spontaneously (without treatment).
B   It will become malignant in approximately 2% of cases.
C   The patient will develop limitation of rotation of the neck to the side of the tumour.
D   The patient can develop neck tilt many years later in spite of initial complete recovery of neck movements.
E   Most patients need surgical treatment.

14.14. Which of the following is/are recognized complications of cavernous haemangioma?

A   Cardiac failure.
B   Local gigantism.
C   Consumptive coagulopathy.
D   Malignant disease.
E   Severe bleeding.

14.15. A port-wine stain in an infant aged 1 month will

A   get worse over the next 1–2 years then regress.
B   indicate a risk of occurrence in 1 in 8 future siblings.
C   remain permanently.
D   probably become malignant if not excised during childhood.
E   respond well to treatment with carbon dioxide snow.

14.16. Which of the following is/are true of haemangiomas?

A   Strawberry naevi are not usually apparent at birth.
B   Strawberry naevi ultimately regress completely.
C   Facial port-wine naevus indicates a risk of seizures.
D   Thrombocytopenia is a recognized complication of haemangioma.
E   Corticosteroid treatment usually causes mixed cavernous capillary haemangiomas to regress.

14.13. A C D

The exact aetiology of the sternomastoid tumour is not known. It is thought to be due to an injury. The tumour resolves spontaneously. Contracture of the muscle occurs. It does not become malignant. There is limitation of the rotation of the neck to the side of the tumour because of the unopposed action of the contracted muscle. The patient may make an apparent recovery but contracture of the sternomastoid may continue which may result in development of a neck tilt subsequently. Most patients recover following neck physiotherapy exercises and do not require surgical treatment.

14.14. A B C

In cavernous haemangioma, cardiac failure occurs because of presence of arteriovenous fistulae, local gigantism is due to increased blood supply and consumptive coagulopathy occurs in haemangiomas because of intravascular coagulation. Malignant disease is rare and severe bleeding does not occur.

14.15. C

A port-wine stain is a mature capillary haemangioma and does not resolve spontaneously. There is no known inheritance and it does not become malignant. Scarring will result if it is treated with carbon dioxide snow.

14.16. A B C D E

Strawberry naevi may not be evident at birth. They tend to grow more rapidly than the infant and may attain large sizes before regressing completely. Facial port-wine naevi are sometimes associated with similar naevi in the meninges (and choroid) resulting in fits due to focal irritation. Cavernous haemangioma trap platelets and cause thrombocytopenia. They regress when treated with corticosteroids.

14.17. Acute osteomyelitis
A   is most commonly situated in the metaphyses of long bones.
B   is unlikely in the presence of a normal X-ray appearance.
C   is most frequently caused by *Staphylococcus aureus*.
D   is often associated with a positive blood culture.
E   is best treated initially with benzyl penicillin while awaiting sensitivity tests.

14.18. The usual form of acute osteomyelitis of the tibia in a child is
A   associated with pain and pyrexia.
B   located in the metaphysis.
C   commonly associated with bacteraemia.
D   commonly associated with mild trauma.
E   treated with penicillin.

14.19. Which of the following is/are appropriate for the management of acute osteomyelitis?
A   Blood culture.
B   CT scan.
C   Bone scan.
D   Strict bed rest.
E   Treatment with amoxycillin.

14.20. Infants presenting with multiple fractures suggest the possibility of
A   active rickets.
B   achondroplasia.
C   osteogenesis imperfecta.
D   non-accidental injury.
E   scurvy.

14.17. A C D
Acute osteomyelitis is due to a blood-borne infection and is situated at the metaphyses at the entrance of the nutrient artery. X-ray changes do not appear for a week after the onset of illness. The commonest organism is *Staphylococcus aureus* followed by *Streptococcus pyogenes* as next commonest. Treatment should be commenced with penicillin and cloxacillin in combination because of the possibility of penicillin-resistant staphylococci.

14.18. A B C D
Acute osteomyelitis is a blood-borne infection in the bone which presents with fever and pain at the site of infection which is usually located in the metaphysis and the entrance of the nutrient artery. Most patients give a history of mild trauma. The treatment of choice is penicillin and cloxacillin because the most common organisms are *Staphylococcus aureus* and *Streptococcus pyogenes*.

14.19. A C
In acute osteomyelitis bone scan shows increased uptake due to hyperaemia. It is very useful in the early diagnosis of acute osteomyelitis. Blood culture is positive in 60% of cases and will be helpful in determining choice of antibiotic. The commonet organism is *Staphylococcus aureus* which may not be sensitive to amoxycillin. Strict bed rest is not indicated.

14.20. C D
Though rickets may cause abnormality of the shape of the bones and greenstick fractures it does not cause complete fractures. In scurvy there is bleeding in the periosteum and dislocation of the costochondral junctions. In osteogenesis imperfecta there is bone fragility which leads to multiple fractures and deformity of the long bones. In non-accidental injury multiple fractures that are at different stages of healing are found. In achondroplasia there is failure of growth of bone at the epiphyseal ends.

14.21. Which of the following complications occur(s) more frequently in association with supracondylar fracture of the humerus than with other limb fractures?
A   Osteomyelitis.
B   Peripheral nerve injury.
C   Volkmann's ischaemic contracture.
D   Fat embolism.
E   Non-union.

14.22. Which of the following is true of infantile seborrhoeic dermatitis?
A   It is seen in first weeks of life.
B   Scalp and flexures are involved.
C   It is often accompanied with candida napkin rash.
D   The skin is usually dry and itchy.
E   It presents with blistering.

14.23. Which of the following conditions can be confused with nappy rash?
A   Moniliasis.
B   Psoriasis.
C   Urinary tract infection.
D   Infantile eczema.
E   Seborrhoeic dermatitis.

14.24. Erythema nodosum can be due to
A   streptococal infection.
B   sarcoid.
C   drug hypersensitivity.
D   Crohn's disease (regional ileitis).
E   Yersinia infection.

14.21. B C
Volkmann's ischaemic contracture is due to disturbance of blood supply to the forearm following supracondylar fractures. The ulnar nerve is involved because of its proximity to the site of the fracture. The other complications can occur equally commonly in any fracture.

14.22. A B C
Seborrhoeic dermatitis in infants usually occurs within the first month of life. The lesions appear in the flexural surfaces and over the scalp. As cradle cap it may be patchy or may spread to almost the entire body. There is usually superadded infection with *Candida albicans*. Lesions are usually non-pruritic. There is no blistering. The presence of weeping lesions with pruritus suggests the possibiilty of coexistent atopic dermatitis.

14.23. A B D E
Moniliasis, psoriasis, infantile eczema and seborrhoeic dermatitis can all be confused with nappy rash. Closer observation of a lesion, e.g. satellite lesions in moniliasis, will establish the correct diagnosis. In urinary tract infection there is no nappy rash.

14.24. A B C D E
Erythema nodosum is due to localized hypersensitivity of the skin to bacterial protein (streptococcus, tubercle bacillus, yersinia) spirochaetes, drugs (iodides, sulphonamides, penicillin) and is also seen in chronic diseases such as sarcoid and Crohn's disease.

14.25. Erythema multiforme is due to

A   drugs.
B   herpes simplex infection.
C   mycoplasma infection.
D   vaccination.
E   post-staphylococcal infection.

14.26. Which of the following conditions remit spontaneously?

A   Hairy naevus.
B   Strawberry naevus.
C   Port-wine stain.
D   Naevus flammeus (stork-bite)
E   Eosinophilic rash (toxic erythema).

14.27. Which of the following is/are characteristic of juvenile rheumatoid arthritis?

A   Unexplained high fever.
B   Morning joint stiffness.
C   Skin rash.
D   Generalized lymphadenopathy.
E   Specific autoantibody.

14.28. Which of the following statements is/are true of Duchenne muscular dystrophy?

A   Antenatal diagnosis can be made.
B   Serum creatine kinase is raised from birth.
C   Sitting up is delayed.
D   The knee jerk becomes depressed before the ankle jerk.
E   At least 10% of affected persons will have mental deficiency.

14.25. A B C D E

Erythema multiforme is characterized by erythematous macules, urticarial lesions, papules, vesicles and bullae. The most characteristic lesion is the target or iris lesion. It is a hypersensitive disorder as a result of immune complexes formed in the body either due to drugs or microbial antigens such as *Herpes simplex*, mycoplasma, vaccinia or staphylococcus.

14.26. B D E

The strawberry naevus enlarges at first and subsequently resolves as it outgrows its blood supply leaving a faint discoloured scar. Eosinophilic rash appears in the neonatal period, the aetiology of which is not clear. It resolves spontaneously. Naevus flammeus is composed of mature capillaries and can fade later in infancy and childhood. Port-wine stains are large naevi flammeus and are permanent. Hairy naevi to not resolve.

14.27. A B C D

Manifestations of juvenile rheumatoid arthritis include unexplained high fever (Still's disease), stiffness of the joints in the morning, skin rash which may be evanescent and generalized lymphadenopathy. Rheumatoid factor may be found but is not specific to rheumatoid arthritis.

14.28. A B D E

In Duchenne muscular dystrophy serum CPK concentration is already elevated at birth and during the preclinical phase. The onset is usually before the age of 4 years but may range from 1 to 10 years. There is no delay in sitting up and the proximal group of muscles are involved before the distal muscles (knee jerk becomes depressed before the ankle jerk). Mental deficiency is a recognized association. If the index case is known, antenatal diagnosis can be made in subsequent siblings by DNA analysis.

14.29. A boy aged 2 years presents with a history of delayed milestones, muscular hypotonia and depressed tendon reflexes. Which of the following statements is/are true?

A A normal serum creatine kinase level (no technical error) excludes the possibility of Duchenne type muscular dystrophy.

B Muscular hypotonia excludes the possibility of cerebral palsy.

C Fasciculation of the tongue would suggest peripheral neuropathy.

D Spinal muscular atrophy is a possible diagnosis.

E Electromyography would be more useful in diagnosing a lower motor neurone cause than a cerebral cause for his problem.

14.30. Which of the following statements is/are true of Duchenne type muscular dystrophy (DMD)?

A Fewer than 50% of affected people live more than 25 years.

B Cardiomyopathy is a recognized feature.

C There is an increased incidence of intellectual handicap.

D The preferred treatment for scoliosis complicating DMD is a Milwaukee brace.

E Investigations can confirm or refute the diagnosis at 1 month of age in babies at risk.

14.29. A D E

In Duchenne muscular dystrophy serum creatine kinase is raised at birth and markedly increased in the initial stages. It is low in established disease. In some forms of cerebral palsy hypotonia is the major feature of the disease. Fasciculation of the tongue suggests involvement of the anterior horn cells. EMG will show decreased potentials with lower motor neurone disease whereas no changes with cerebral problems. Spinal muscular atrophy is a possible diagnosis.

14.30. A B C E

Death due to Duchenne muscular dystrophy occurs in more than 75% of cases before the age of 20 years. The majority of patients have cardiomyopathy which is the chief cause of death. The mean IQ of children with Duchenne muscular dystrophy is 80; 25% have frank mental deficiency. Serum creatine kinase values are increased even at birth in these patients. No treatment (orthopaedic or Milwaukee brace) is recommended as it will make the patient less ambulant and predispose to pneumonia.

15 Drugs, accidents and poisoning

15.1. Which of the following statements is/are true of paracetamol?
A   It has no anti-inflammatory action.
B   It has been implicated in the causation of Reye's syndrome.
C   Toxic doses are known to cause hepatic failure.
D   It is the drug of choice for infants with fever.
E   It is contraindicated in patients with history of asthma.

15.2. Tricyclic antidepressants are useful in the treatment of
A   enuresis.
B   encopresis.
C   endogenous depression.
D   nightmares.
E   emotional deprivation.

15.3. Which of the following is/are true of sodium cromoglycate?
A   It is a bronchodilator.
B   It inhibits the release of mediators of the allergic reaction from the cells.
C   It is only useful in atopic individuals.
D   It is useful in children with exercise-induced asthma.
E   Therapy should be given during episodes of severe asthma.

15.4. Phenobarbitone
A   is known to cause agitation and hyperactivity in children.
B   has been shown to be effective prophylaxis in recurrent febrile convulsions.
C   is contraindicated for neonatal seizures.
D   has a half life of more than 12 hours.
E   may interfere with a child's cognitive performance.

15.1. A C D

Paracetamol has analgesic and antipyretic activity but no anti-inflammatory action. It is excreted in the urine after conjugation to glucuronide or sulphate by liver. Toxic symptoms include vomiting, hypotension and sweating. Liver damage occurs after ingestion of large doses (15 g). Reye's syndrome or analgesic nephropathy have not been recorded following treatment with paracetamol. It does not exacerbate symptoms of asthma.

15.2. A C

Indications for the use of tricylcic antidepressants are depression, nocturnal enuresis and chronic intractable pain. It has not been shown to be of any use in encopresis, nightmares or emotional deprivation. Contraindications are hypersensitivity and simultaneous administration of monoamine oxidase inhibitors. It should be used with caution in epilepsy, cardiovascular disease, heart block, glaucoma, hyperthyroidism and urinary obstruction because of its anticholinergic effect.

15.3. B D

Sodium cromoglycate inhibits the release from sensitized cells of mediators of the allergic reaction, viz. it inhibits the degranulation of mast cells which prevents both the immediate and the late asthmatic response to immunological and other stimuli. Given regular prophylaxis it is useful in all forms of asthma including that due to exercise. It is not a bronchodilator and is of no use during an acute severe asthmatic attack.

15.4. A B D E

Phenobarbitone is a long-acting barbiturate because of its slow metabolism which results in a half-life of more than 12 hours. Besides sodium valproate it is the only drug that is effective prophylaxis for recurrent febrile convulsions though it has a disadvantage of causing hyperactivity in some children and may interfere with the child's cognitive performance. It is the first-line drug for treatment of neonatal seizures though it is not very effective in hypoxic-ischaemic encephalopathy.

15.5. Which of the following statements is/are true?

A The use of antibiotics in otitis media has reduced the incidence of intracranial infection.
B Ampicillin may cause a fine macular rash which is of no clinical significance.
C Tetracyclines are useful in young children.
D Erythromycin may be helpful in mycoplasma infections.
E Penicillin is extracted from a rain forest plant.

15.6. Tetracycline is contraindicated in young children because it causes

A bulging fontanelle.
B gastrointestinal disturbance.
C cholestatic jaundice.
D inhibition of vitamin K synthesis.
E dental discoloration.

15.7. Recognized side effects of phenytoin (Dilantin) administration include

A ataxia.
B hirsutism.
C hypertrophy of the gums.
D lymphadenopathy.
E renal papillary necrosis.

15.8. Which of the following is/are true of methylxanthines (theophylline)?

A The slow-release preparations are predictably absorbed from the gastrointestinal tract regardless of presence of food.
B Pharmacokinetics of the drugs vary considerably from patient to patient.
C They cause stimulation of the central nervous system.
D They stimulate intracellular adenyl cyclase production.
E They are not universally well tolerated by children.

15.5 A B D
Antibiotic treatment of otitis media has reduced the incidence of mastoiditis and spread of infection to the brain. A fine macular rash which is not itchy sometimes occurs following administration of ampicillin. It resolves within a short time and does not indicate allergy. Tetracyclines cause discoloration of the teeth and are not recommended for treatment of children. Erythromycin has been demonstrated to be effective in treatment of mycoplasma infections. Penicillin was originally derived from a mould. Most penicillins are now synthesized.

15.6. E
Tetracyclines are deposited in the teeth and bones. They cause discoloration of teeth in children. In young infants they can cause bulging fontanelle. Cholestatic jaundice is not a feature of tetracycline therapy.

15.7. A B C D
The side effects of phenytoin (Dilantin) include central nervous system manifestations (nystagmus, ataxia, mental confusion), gastrointestinal symptoms (nausea, vomiting and constipation), skin rashes varying from a mild rash to Stevens–Johnson's syndrome, bone marrow depression and lymphadenopathy, hirsutism and gingival hypertrophy.

15.8. B C E
The absorption of slow-release preparations of theophylline is altered when they are administered with a meal and may be accelerated or delayed depending upon the product. The pharmokinetics of the drugs vary considerably from patient to patient and therefore monitoring of blood levels is important. Many children have severe gastrointestinal symptoms and central nervous system stimulation which prevents their administration in such children. Intracellular adenyl cyclase production has not been demonstrated with the adminstration of theophylline.

15.9. Which of the following is/are true of penicillin?
A   They penetrate uninflamed meninges.
B   Phenoxy-methyl penicillin (penicillin V) has the same spectrum of activity as benzylpenicillin.
C   They are recommended as prophylaxis for contacts of meningococcal meningitis.
D   There is no advantage of amoxycillin over ampicillin when given intravenously.
E   Ampicillin need not be discontinued if the patient develops a nonspecific (macular) rash.

15.10. Which of the following statements is/are true of digoxin therapy?
A   It is the drug of choice for treatment of congestive cardiac failure in newborn infants.
B   Hypokalaemia potentiates its toxicity.
C   A high serum digoxin level indicates digoxin toxicity.
D   Anorexia (poor feeding) may be the only symptom of toxicity.
E   Serum digoxin levels should not be measured less than 4 hours after the last dose.

15.11. In which of the following infections is erythromycin a suitable antibiotic?
A   Impetigo.
B   Urinary tract infection.
C   Mycoplasma pneumonia.
D   Campylobacter enteritis.
E   Chlamydia conjunctivitis.

15.12. Beta-blocking agents such as propranolol are contraindicated in the presence of
A   tetralogy of Fallot.
B   hypertrophic obstructive cardiomyopathy.
C   digoxin overdose.
D   asthma.
E   cyanotic congenital heart disease.

15.9. B D E
Though penicillins are found in therapeutic levels in the CSF in the treatment of acute meningitis, they penetrate poorly the uninflamed meninges. The therapeutic activity of phenoxy-methyl penicillin and penicillin is the same though differences in efficacy may occur because of the different blood levels that may be achieved. Many meningococci may be resistant to penicillin and therefore rifampicin is the drug of choice for prophylaxis for contacts of meningococcal meningitis. The spectrum of amoxyllin and ampicillin is the same; the advantage of amoxyllin over ampicillin when given orally is that the peak levels are much higher. The macular rash without itchiness that appears following administration of ampicillin is not allergic and does not require discontinuation of the drug.

15.10. B D E
The drug of choice for treatment of congestive cardiac failure in newborn infants is frusemide (and other diuretics). Hypokalaemia potentiates the toxicity of digoxin. Toxic effects of digoxin include cardiac arrhythmias and anorexia. The absorption of digoxin does not occur for at least 4 hours after administration and hence drug levels should be assessed at least 4 hours after the last dose. Drug levels are useful to determine whether adequate amounts of digoxin are being given rather than establish digoxin toxicity.

15.11. A C D E
Organisms that are sensitive to erythromycin include streptococcal (which causes impetigo), pneumococci, staphylococci, gonococci, *Mycoplasma pneumoniae*, campylobacter and chlamydia. Urinary tract infections are usually caused by Gram-negative organisms which are not sensitive to erythromycin.

15.12. D
Propranolol is a beta-adreno receptor blocking agent which reduces the influence of excessive sympathetic nervous stimulation of the heart reducing pulse rate, blood pressure, cardiac contraction and cardiac output. These effects are of therapeutic value in several cardiovascular diseases including tetralogy of Fallot, hypertrophic obstructive cardiomyopathy and cyanotic congenital heart disease. It is contraindicated in asthma, patients receiving hypoglycaemic agents or verapamil and in congestive heart failure.

15.13. Which of the following have a cause and effect relationship?
A   Polyuria and vitamin D intoxication.
B   Renal stones and vitamin B intoxication.
C   Thalidomide and fetal embryopathy.
D   Visual problems and vitamin A intoxication.
E   Cigarette smoking and intra-uterine growth retardation.

15.14. In cases of severe hypothermia
A   rapid warming is potentially dangerous.
B   the ECG may show a characteristic shortening of PR interval.
C   warming is followed by a metabolic acidosis.
D   plasma cortisol is reduced.
E   hypoglycaemia during rewarming may occur.

15.15. Which of the following is/are associated with salicylate poisoning?
A   Fever.
B   Metabolic acidosis.
C   Respiratory alkalosis.
D   Pin point pupils.
E   Hyperglycaemia.

15.16. Which of the following statements is/are true of childhood accidents?
A   In developed countries they are the commonest cause of death in children after the age of 1 year.
B   They are preventable in the majority of cases.
C   They do not occur in children below the age of 6 months.
D   Protection of the child is the ultimate solution in their prevention.
E   Family social-pathology would account for most accidents in children under 2 years of age.

15.13. A C E

Polyuria in vitamin D intoxication is due to hypercalciuria secondary to hypercalcaemia. Thalidomide causes fetal embryopathy by sensory neuropathy. Epidemiological studies have shown intrauterine growth retardation in mothers who smoke. Vitamin B has not been shown to cause any toxic effects. Vitamin A deficiency causes visual problems, excess causes enlargement of liver and spleen, swelling and pain of long bones, bone fragility and increased intracranial pressure.

15.14. A C E

Rapid warming following severe hypothermia will cause vasodilatation and circulatory failure. Hypoglycaemia results from the rapid use of the glucose and glycogen for the maintenance of body temperature. The metabolic acidosis is the result of the 'oxygen debt'. There are no characteristic ECG changes in severe hypothermia. The plasma cortisone levels are increased.

15.15. A B C E

Salicylates directly stimulate the respiratory centre causing respiratory alkalosis. This is followed by dehydration, hypokalaemia and progressive accumulation of lactic acid and other metabolites resulting in a metabolic acidosis. Both hyperglycaemia and hypoglycaemia have been observed in severe cases. Fever has been observed.

15.16. A B E

Epidemiological studies have shown that accidents are the commonest cause of death after the age of 1 year in developed countries and the majority of them are preventable. In the majority of cases in children under the age of 2 years, accidents are due to disturbed family discord, another sick child, house moving etc. Children under the age of 6 months may fall from 'change tables' or roll over in an unprotected cot. In the younger child protection but in the older child education is the solution in the prevention of accidents.

15.17. Which of the following statements is/are true of burns in children?

A   In developed countries burns are the leading cause of death in the home in children 1–4 years of age.

B   Loss of fluid, electrolytes and protein occurs into the interstitium of both injured and uninjured tissues.

C   Albumin should be administered as soon as possible.

D   Gastric ulcers are usually present in those patients who die.

E   Patients with low urine output need diuretic therapy.

15.18. Which of the following statements about sudden unexpected infant death is/are true?

A   More common in summer.

B   Most common between 2 and 4 months of age.

C   More common among males than females.

D   The commonest cause of death in developed countries between 1 and 12 months.

E   More common among infants that were of low birth weight.

15.19. Sudden infant death syndrome

A   can be diagnosed without a post-mortem.

B   affects all social groups equally.

C   does not occur after the age of 6 months.

D   usually attributable to child abuse.

E   is often preceded by mild upper respiratory tract illness.

15.17. A B D

Accidents in the home (of which burns are most common) are the chief cause of death in children between the age of 1–4 years. Fluid, electrolytes and protein move into the interstitium of injured and uninjured tissues ('third' space) resulting in shock and electrolyte imbalance. Administration of colloids (including albumin) should be withheld for 12–36 hours when the capillary permeability of the injured area returns to normal. Gastrointestinal complications include stress ulcer and perforation. The ulcers are almost universally present in those patients who die. Low urinary output is due to inadequate fluid therapy.

15.18. B C D E

Epidemiological studies have shown that sudden infant deaths (SIDS) occur most commonly between the age of 2–4 months during winter, in males, in prone position and low birth-weight infants. They are the commonest cause of death in developed countries between 1 and 12 months.

15.19. E

The diagnosis of sudden infant death syndrome is one of exclusion and therefore cannot be established without a post-mortem. Epidemiological studies have shown that the incidence is higher in lower socio-economic groups. Sudden infant deaths do occur after the age of 6 months. Many infants give a history of a mild upper respiratory tract infection. By definition sudden infant death syndrome is not due to child abuse.